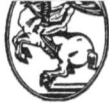

# VIROLOGY MONOGRAPHS

# DIE VIRUSFORSCHUNG IN EINZELDARSTELLUNGEN

CONTINUATION OF / FORTFÜHRUNG VON
HANDBOOK OF VIRUS RESEARCH
HANDBUCH DER VIRUSFORSCHUNG
FOUNDED BY / BEGRÜNDET VON
R. DOERR

EDITED BY / HERAUSGEGEBEN VON
S. GARD · C. HALLAUER

13

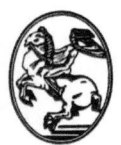

1975
SPRINGER-VERLAG
WIEN NEW YORK

# LACTIC DEHYDROGENASE VIRUS

BY

K. E. K. ROWSON AND B. W. J. MAHY

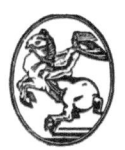

1975

**SPRINGER-VERLAG**

WIEN   NEW YORK

Library of Congress Cataloging in Publication Data. Rowson, K. E. K. 1924–. Lactic dehydrogenase virus. (Virology monographs; 13). 1. Lactic dehydrogenase virus. I. Mahy, Brian W. J., joint author. II. Title. III. Series. [DNLM: 1. Vertebrate viruses, Unclassified. W1 VI83 v. 13 / QW160.V5 R885L]. QR360.V52 no. 13 [QR303]. 599′.3233. 74-34231.

ISBN-13:978-3-7091-8380-9     e-ISBN-13:978-3-7091-8378-6
DOI: 10.1007/978-3-7091-8378-6

# Lactic Dehydrogenase Virus

By

## K. E. K. Rowson

Department of Pathology and Bacteriology,
The Institute of Laryngology and Otology, University of London,
330/332, Gray's Inn Road, London, WC1X 8EE, England

and

## B. W. J. Mahy

Division of Virology, Department of Pathology,
University of Cambridge, Laboratories Block, Addenbrookes Hospital, Hills Road,
Cambridge CB2 2QQ, England

With 54 Figures

## Table of Contents

We wish to express our thanks to our many colleagues who generously provided us
with preprints of their work, and unpublished observations. We are particularly
indebted to those who donated prints of their electron micrographs of the virus.

# I. Introduction

Inapparent virus infections of experimental animals and tissue culture systems
present to the investigator a problem which it is impossible to overcome completely.
Although all recognised viruses can be excluded from an experimental system,
previously unsuspected viruses causing no obvious effects ('silent' viruses) will
continue to be discovered. A truly silent virus would replicate, causing no change
in its host cell, damage to infected tissue or immune response and would presumably be of no consequence. It is the relatively silent viruses which cause virtually no pathological changes but can alter the response of a test system, which are
important. The lactic dehydrogenase virus (LDV) is an interesting example of
such a virus. It causes no clinical disease in mice but can significantly alter their
response to other infective agents and to the development of tumours. If the ideal
virus is one which replicates rapidly and continuously without killing its host and
is easily transmitted, LDV must be almost perfect. It replicates very rapidly in
mice of all strains so far tested, produces a stable infection with a continuously high
level of infective virus in the blood for the remainder of the animal's life, yet causes
no harm to its host. It lacks, however, one important property; the ability to pass
readily from one animal to another under natural conditions. Infected females
often fail to infect their young and transmission between adults is not very frequent. However, no doubt because of the permanence of the infected state, the
virus survives in wild mice and is easily transmitted inadvertently by experimental procedures. Any tissue taken from an infected mouse will be highly
infectious, and this has resulted in many viruses and tumours passed in mice
being contaminated with LDV.

The detection of silent virus infections is often quite simple once a test system has been described. It is interesting that LDV was discovered independently in three laboratories at about the same time, but detected by entirely different methods in each case. The first method to be reported and the most useful way of diagnosing the infection was that described by RILEY and his colleagues (RILEY, LILLY, HUERTO, and BARDELL, 1960), namely a massive increase in the level of lactate dehydrogenase (LDH) activity in the plasma of infected mice. In the other two laboratories, infection with LDV was recognized by less specific methods: in one by a moderate degree of splenomegaly (POPE, 1961) and in the other by interference with the replication of vesicular stomatitis virus (ROWE, HARTLEY, and HUEBNER, 1962).

RILEY's discovery of LDV resulted from the study of plasma enzyme levels in tumour-bearing experimental animals. The levels of activity of a number of plasma enzymes had proved useful in the diagnosis and follow-up of certain disease processes including some tumours (WILKINSON, 1962). For example, acid phosphatase activity was raised in patients with carcinoma of the prostate (GUTMAN and GUTMAN, 1938) and alkaline phosphatase in cases of osteogenic sarcoma (FRANSEEN and MCLEAN, 1941). In a search for further tests which could be used in the early diagnosis of tumours, plasma enzyme levels were measured in tumour-bearing experimental animals and patients. Plasma aldolase levels were found to be raised in tumour-bearing rats and in 20 per cent of patients with cancer (SIBLEY and LEHNINGER, 1949, a and b) and plasma LDH levels in patients with a number of different malignant tumours (HILL and LEVI, 1954). In mice bearing a transplantable rhabdomyosarcoma, the plasma LDH level showed a sharp rise by the fourth day after implantation. The plasma LDH activity remained elevated but showed no further rise until tumour growth had become extensive when a further rise in LDH activity was observed (HSIEH, SUNTZEFF, and COWDRY, 1956). WRÓBLEWSKI and LA DUE (1955) found that the plasma LDH level was raised in patients with myocardial infarction and in cases of leukaemia of the acute stem cell and chronic myelogenous types. FRIEND and WRÓBLEWSKI (1956) followed up this observation by observing the plasma LDH level in mice injected with four transplantable strains of murine leukaemia. The strains varied in their speed of growth and in the length of time the recipient mice survived. The rapidly growing strains caused a rapid and progressive rise in plasma LDH activity but the most slowly growing strains which took 17 days to kill the mice caused a biphasic rise in plasma LDH activity similar to the changes reported previously by HSIEH, SUNTZEFF, and COWDRY (1956) using the transplantable rhabdomyosarcoma. A similar early rise in plasma LDH occurring within 3 days of injection of tumour cells was reported by MANSO, SUGIURA, and WRÓBLEWSKI (1958). RILEY and WRÓBLEWSKI (1960) examined in greater detail the plasma LDH changes following the injection of mice with Ehrlich carcinoma cells. They observed 5 phases in the plasma LDH curves from the tumour-bearing mice (Fig. 1). There was a latent period of 1 to 2 days after tumour implantation followed by a rapid increase in enzyme activity from normal values of approximately 500 units to between 2,000 and 6,000 units. This 5- to 10-fold increase occurred before detectable tumour growth could be observed and was followed by a plateau level of LDH activity for several days before a second rapid rise occurred as the tumour enlarged.

With increasing tumour mass plasma LDH activity rose to a level of 25,000 to 50,000 units. The final phase was a fall in plasma LDH activity just prior to death. RILEY and WRÓBLEWSKI (1960) treated mice bearing Ehrlich carcinomas with orthophenylenediamine, an anti-tumour drug, and noted that as the tumour regressed, the plasma LDH level fell but although some of the mice remained tumour-free for several months, the plasma enzyme activity never returned to a completely normal level. In further experiments, RILEY and his co-workers (RILEY,

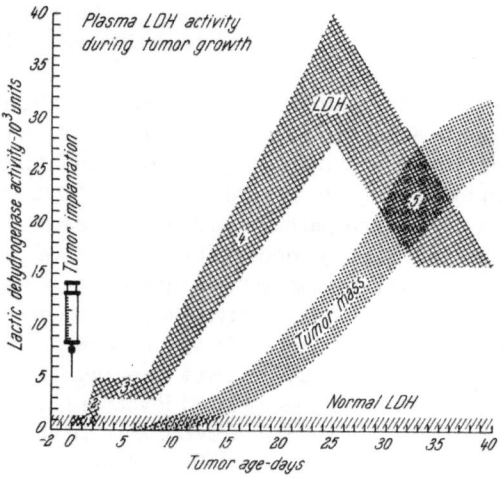

Fig. 1. Correlation of the five phases of lactic dehydrogenase (LDH) activity in the plasma with progressive growth of the solid Ehrlich carcinoma in mice.
The complex enzyme response following tumour implantation is due to the combined effect of infection with LDV and tumour growth. (From RILEY and WRÓBLEWSKI, 1960)

LILLY, HUERTO, and BARDELL, 1960) found that the injection of plasma from tumour bearing mice into normal mice caused an early rise in plasma LDH activity which occurred within 3 days and was similar in magnitude to the early rise in LDH activity following the transplantation of tumour tissue. The 5- to 10-fold increase in plasma LDH activity caused in this way was permanent, although the mice did not develop tumours and, what was even more remarkable, the alteration in plasma LDH activity could be transmitted serially from mouse to mouse by the injection of plasma or tissue extracts. An infective agent was clearly responsible for the raised plasma LDH activity and its presence in the plasma of infected mice was stable and permanent. The causative agent was inactivated by heating to 70° C and would pass through bacteria-proof filters. It was, therefore, a virus-size particle and appeared to be responsible for the early rise in plasma LDH activity which had been observed previously by workers using transplantable murine tumours and leukaemia. Figure 2 shows the plasma LDH levels in mice injected with leukaemia cells contaminated with LDV or free of the virus, and the response to the virus alone. It is clear that the biphasic response is due to the combined action of LDV and the tumour cells. RILEY and his co-workers (RILEY, LILLY, HUERTO, and BARDELL, 1960) examined 26 transplantable murine tumours and found the virus in each of them. This suggested that the virus might play some part in the neoplastic process but it soon became clear that it was a chance contaminant of any tumour or virus preparation passed in mice. It was not present in the plasma of mice with primary tumours either spontaneous (MUNDY and WILLIAMS, 1961; NOTKINS, BERRY, MOLONEY, and GREENFIELD, 1962; GEORGII, BAYERLE, BRDICZKA, and ZOBL, 1963), or induced by X-rays or chemical carcinogens (RILEY, 1961 and

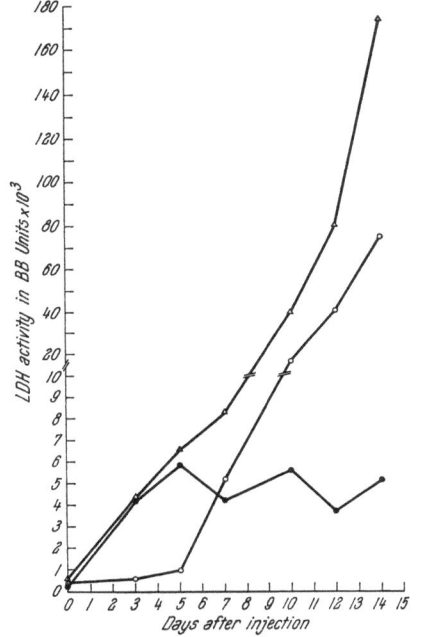

Fig. 2. Plasma lactic dehydrogenase activity in AKR mice following the injection of leukaemic cells contaminated with LDV (△———△) or free of the virus (○———○) and LDV alone (●———●). (From ADAMS, ROWSON, and SALAMAN, 1961)

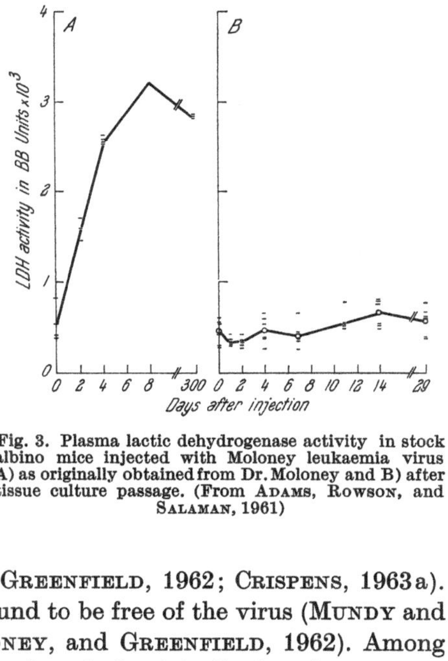

Fig. 3. Plasma lactic dehydrogenase activity in stock albino mice injected with Moloney leukaemia virus A) as originally obtained from Dr. Moloney and B) after tissue culture passage. (From ADAMS, ROWSON, and SALAMAN, 1961)

1962b; NOTKINS, BERRY, MOLONEY, and GREENFIELD, 1962; CRISPENS, 1963a). A few transplantable tumours were also found to be free of the virus (MUNDY and WILLIAMS, 1961; NOTKINS, BERRY, MOLONEY, and GREENFIELD, 1962). Among the 26 tumours which RILEY and his co-workers had originally found to contain the virus were leukaemias induced by the Friend and Moloney leukaemia viruses. These viruses were shown to be contaminated with LDV (ADAMS, ROWSON, and SALAMAN, 1961; MAHY, ROWSON, SALAMAN, and PARR, 1964; NOTKINS, BERRY, MOLONEY, and GREENFIELD, 1962). When these leukaemia viruses were passed through mouse embryo tissue cultures or newborn rats, the LDH virus was lost and the purified leukaemia viruses no longer caused a rise in plasma LDH activity before the development of advanced leukaemia (Fig. 3).

In spite of the large amount of virus produced and evidence that the activity of the reticuloendothelial system was impaired in LDV-infected mice (MAHY, 1964), no histological changes were readily detected (RILEY, HUERTO, BARDELL, LOVE-

LESS, and FITZMAURICE, 1962). However, it has recently been shown that there is necrosis of thymic-dependent areas in the spleen and lymph nodes during the first 48 hours after infection followed by proliferation of germinal centre cells resulting in a minor degree of splenomegaly (PROFFITT and CONGDON, 1970; PROF-FITT, CONGDON, and TYNDALL, 1972; SNODGRASS and HANNA, 1970; SNODGRASS, LOWREY, and HANNA, 1972; SANTISTEBAN, RILEY, and FITZMAURICE, 1972). It was this increase in spleen weight in mice inoculated with a saline suspension of liver and spleen from a wild house mouse which led POPE (1961) to suspect the presence of a virus he designated WMI. This virus which was maintained by serial passage in mice was subsequently shown to have identical properties to LDV (POPE and ROWE, 1964). Antigenic identity between the two viruses could not be demonstrated because although antibodies are produced in infected mice, they only incompletely inactivate viral infectivity. The failure of antisera to neutralize the virus accounts for the permanent viraemia and is one of the most interesting features of infection with LDV.

The altered response of mice infected with LDV to other infective agents, tumours and therapeutic procedures, causes the virus to be of importance to anyone working with experimental mice (ALLISON, 1963; RILEY, 1962b; EBERT, CHIRIGOS, and CHAN, 1970; RILEY, 1974b and c; RILEY and SPECKMAN, 1974). It was the interfering ability of LDV contaminating preparations of Moloney leukaemia virus which led ROWE and his colleagues (ROWE, HARTLEY, and HUEBNER, 1962; ROWE, 1963) to recognise its presence. They were trying to develop a method of titrating Moloney leukaemia virus on the hypothesis that it might induce interference in suckling mice against a lethal virus susceptible to interference. Vesicular stomatitis virus was chosen and filtrates of Moloney leu-kaemia were found to have a very marked interfering ability against this virus. Thus, it at first appeared that they had found a method of titrating Moloney leukaemia virus but further investigation showed that it was not the Moloney virus in-ducing the interference but a new virus which proved to be identical with LDV.

The induction of tumours by chemical carcinogens or X-rays has not been shown to be consistently affected by the presence of LDV but the development of mammary tumours in mice appears to be delayed in LDV-infected animals (RILEY, 1966a). An interesting example of the way in which the accidental presence of LDV can affect an experiment is to be seen in the testing of arginase as a therapeutic agent in mouse leukaemia. The transplantable leukaemic cells used were contami-nated with the LDV which, because it blocked the clearance of arginase from the plasma, markedly potentiated the action of the enzyme and gave a false impression of the potency of the enzyme in uninfected animals (RILEY, 1968a, 1970).

The LDV-infected mouse has a permanent viraemia and impaired function of the reticuloendothelial system, which results in grossly abnormal plasma enzyme levels. The mouse produces antibodies to the virus which fail to inactivate it, yet the animal remains in perfect health. One might have expected such a unique infection to have attracted a large group of workers from many disciplines, but in fact comparatively little interest has been taken in LDV. This is probably because the virus has not proved readily amenable to quantitative study in vitro. An additional reason could be that the infection is confined to the mouse as a species, and no obvious counterpart has so far been described in humans. However, a number of important clinical diseases are probably related to inapparent ('slow') virus infections (PORTER, 1971; LEADER and HURVITZ, 1972) and further study of the interaction of LDV with its host could provide valuable information on the ecology of inapparent infections in general. There have been six previous reviews: GEORGII (1964); NOTKINS (1965a); RILEY (1966b); BENDINELLI (1967); RILEY (1968b); RILEY (1974a).

## II. Classification and Nomenclature

RILEY and his colleagues (RILEY, LILLY, HUERTO, and BARDELL, 1960) found that mice injected with plasma from mice bearing certain transplantable tumours developed a ten-fold or greater rise in plasma LDH activity within 3 days and that this alteration in plasma enzyme level could be serially transmitted from one mouse to another by some agent in the plasma. They thus demonstrated that they were dealing with an infective agent. They also showed that the agent was small enough to pass through a bacteria-proof filter. Later filtration experiments (ROWSON, MAHY, and SALAMAN, 1963) showed that the diameter of the infective particle was approximately 45 nm. It was therefore a virus.

Table 1. *Synonyms for Lactic Dehydrogenase Virus*

| Name used | Reference |
|---|---|
| Enzyme elevating factor | RILEY, LILLY, HUERTO and BARDELL (1960) |
| Lactate dehydrogenase virus | CRISPENS (1966a) |
| Lactic dehydrogenase agent | BAILEY, STEARMAN and CLOUGH (1963) |
| Lactic dehydrogenase-augmenting agent | YAFFE (1962a) |
| Lactic dehydrogenase elevating virus | ROWSON, ADAMS and SALAMAN (1961) |
| Lactic dehydrogenase factor | NOTKINS, BERRY, MOLONEY and GREENFIELD (1962) |
| Lactic dehydrogenase virus | NOTKINS (1965a) |
| Plasma lactic dehydrogenase-elevating virus | PLAGEMANN, WATANABE and SWIM (1962) |
| Riley agent | ADAMS, ROWSON and SALAMAN (1961) |
| Riley virus | ADAMS, ROWSON and SALAMAN (1961) |
| Riley's enzyme elevating virus | ROWSON, ADAMS and SALAMAN (1962) |
| Riley's lactic dehydrogenase virus | WILNER (1969) |
| Riley's plasma enzyme elevating virus | MAHY (1964) |

Various names have been used by different authors for this virus (see Table 1) but the one in most common use is lactic dehydrogenase virus and this name will be used in the present review. The name can be criticized on the grounds that other enzymes besides LDH also show increased levels of activity in mice infected with the virus and that lactic dehydrogenase should now be called lactate dehydrogenase (E.C.1.1.1.27). However, MELNICK (1971), WILNER (1969) and ANDREWES and PEREIRA (1972) in their classifications of animal viruses use the name lactic dehydrogenase virus. The International Committee on Nomenclature of Viruses in their first report (WILDY, 1971) suggest the use of a hierarchical system of classification with latinized binomial nomenclature, but such a system is widely regarded as unsatisfactory for bacteria and viruses (GIBBS, HARRISON, WATSON, and WILDY, 1966). In any case, no doubt because of lack of data on the structure of LDV and its nucleic acid, the International Committee in their report did not assign LDV to one of the 43 groups of viruses which they defined.

Several authors have drawn attention to similarities between LDV and other viruses. CRISPENS (1965a) and TENNANT (1966) independently noted similarities between LDV and three other mouse viruses: pneumonia virus of mice, mouse hepatitis virus and lymphocytic choriomeningitis virus. These four viruses are of medium size, ether sensitive, heat labile, contain RNA, produce no cytopathic effect in tissue cultures, and with the exception of the pneumonia virus do not agglutinate erythrocytes. However, more recent work suggests that pneumonia virus of mice is a metamyxovirus (MELNICK, 1971) and that mouse hepatitis and lymphocytic choriomeningitis viruses are more closely related to other viruses than to LDV. Mouse hepatitis virus has now been placed with avian infectious bronchitis virus and certain human respiratory viruses in the coronavirus group (ALMEIDA et al., 1968) and lymphocytic choriomeningitis virus has been shown to be very similar in structure and to share antigens with the Tacaribe subgroup of arboviruses. For these arboviruses the name arenovirus has been proposed (ROWE et al., 1970).

Electron microscopy of thin sections of LDV preparations has revealed elliptical or oblong particles 36 to 42 nm wide and 45 to 75 nm long (DE THÉ and NOTKINS, 1965). If, in fact, the virus is oblong it would be unique among the viruses of vertebrates so far studied (FENNER, 1968). Bee chronic paralysis is an oblong RNA virus but GIBBS (1969) found that LDV was larger, had particles of only one size, had a larger sedimentation coefficient and was disrupted by treatment with ether. It thus seems unlikely that LDV is related to bee chronic paralysis virus. LDV appears to be most closely related to rubella virus and the arboviruses of groups A and B. All these viruses are of the same size and shape and possess a lipid-containing envelope. The name togavirus has been proposed for the group (MELNICK, 1971; ANDREWES et al., 1970). The fine structure of one member, Sindbis virus, has been investigated after removal of the outer envelope with sodium deoxycholate (HORZINEK and MUSSGAY, 1969). The viral nucleocapsid was 35 nm in diameter and composed of 32 capsomeres. However, published electron micrographs of LDV (see p. 14) are not sufficiently good to reveal detailed fine structure and until more data is available the possible relationship of LDV to the togavirus group must remain in doubt (HORZINEK, 1973). Recently, ALMEIDA and MIMS (1974) using immune electron microscopy have obtained pictures of LDV particles showing distinct morphological differences between LDV and togaviruses of group B. The particles in their pictures have a bottle-shaped morphology and they propose that the descriptive name "lagenavirus" be applied to LDV and any other viruses found to have a similar morphology.

# III. Isolation, Purification, and Titration

The LDV replicates rapidly on injection into mice and causes a sudden and permanent rise in the plasma LDH activity. Figure 4 shows the infective virus titre and level of LDH activity in the blood of mice following the injection of LDV. The titre commences to rise six hours after infection and reaches a peak level after

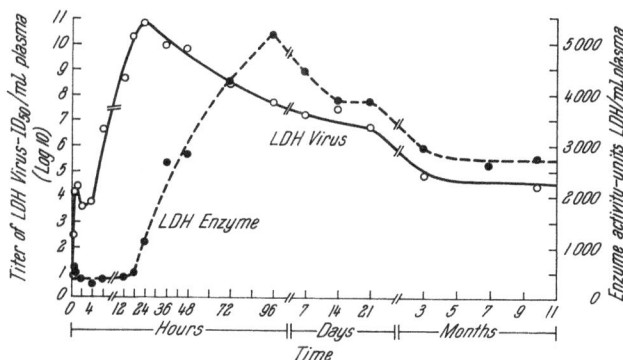

Fig. 4. Plasma lactic dehydrogenase activity and titre of LDV in the plasma of mice following injection of LDV. (From NOTKINS and SHOCHAT, 1963)

twenty-four hours. The LDH activity does not rise until 18 hours after infection and reaches a maximum level after 3—4 days. Both the virus titre and LDH activity in the plasma fall slowly from their peak values over the course of a week or more to reach stable levels where they remain remarkably constant for months, the LDH activity some 5 to 10 times the normal and the virus titre $10^4$ $ID_{50}$ per ml of plasma. Figure 5 shows the change in plasma LDH activity following the injection of different doses of virus. The LDH level rises more rapidly in the mice receiving the larger dose of virus, but by 3 days after infection, the LDH activity is virtually the same regardless of the dose of virus injected. Mice which do not show the characteristic rise in plasma LDH activity three days after injection of test material may safely be assumed not to have been infected as their plasma LDH level will not subsequently rise and they remain normally susceptible to infection with the virus. The fact that the plasma enzyme response is independent of the infecting dose of virus is not surprising in view of the rapidity with which virus replication occurs after infection.

The rise in plasma enzyme activity is for practical purposes the only way of detecting infection with LDV as infected mice remain in perfect health. The only pathological changes which have been noted are a very minor enlargement of the spleen (see p. 91) and impairment of function of the reticuloendothelial system (see p. 72).

LDV is readily isolated by the injection of infected material into mice of any strain. No difference in strain susceptibility has been reported but SJL/J mice show a greater rise in plasma LDH level than other strains (CRISPENS, 1971). This appears to be due to the level of activity of the reticuloendothelial system and is a

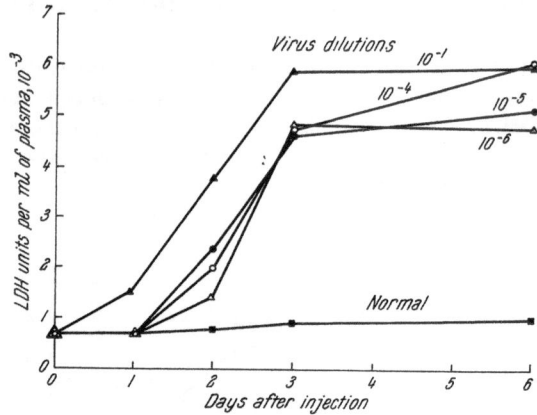

Fig. 5. Plasma lactic dehydrogenase activity in mice following the injection of different doses of LDV. Each point is the mean level in a group of 5 mice. Each mouse received 0.1 ml intraperitoneally of the indicated dilutions of mouse plasma from an infected mouse. (From PLAGEMANN, GREGORY, SWIM, and CHAN, 1963)

Table 2. *Mouse Strains in which Lactic Dehydrogenase Virus has been Found to Replicate*

| Mouse strain | Reference |
|---|---|
| A | MUNDY and WILLIAMS (1961) |
| AKR | ADAMS, ROWSON and SALAMAN (1961) |
| BALB/c | BAILEY, STEARMAN and CLOUGH (1963) |
| BR 6 | MUNDY and WILLIAMS (1961) |
| C 57/Bl | YAFFE (1962) |
| CAF-1 | NOTKINS and GREENFIELD (1962) |
| CBA | ADAMS, ROWSON and SALAMAN (1961) |
| CDF 1 | DU BUY and JOHNSON (1965) |
| CFW | PLAGEMANN, WATANABE and SWIM (1962) |
| C 3 H | CRISPENS (1963a) |
| DBA/2 | NOTKINS, BERRY, MOLONEY and GREENFIELD (1962) |
| LCS/Fg | CRISPENS (1966b) |
| NMRI | GEORGII, LENZ and ZOBEL (1964) |
| QIMR | POPE and ROWE (1964) |
| SIM/McK | STEERES, MIRAND, THOMSON and AVILA (1969) |
| SJL/J | CRISPENS (1971) |
| Swiss ICR | RILEY, LILLY, HUERTO and BARDELL (1960) |
| SWR/J | OLDSTONE and DIXON (1971) |
| Stock albino strain (Schofield) | ADAMS, ROWSON and SALAMAN (1961) |

recessive trait under the control of a single gene at an autosomal locus (CRISPENS, 1972). Table 2 gives a list of the various strains which have been used and reported in the literature. Mice are susceptible to infection by parenteral injection of infected material by any route. Two characteristics of LDV are sufficiently unique to be considered definitive for identification:

(i) a 5- to 10-fold elevation of plasma LDH activity occurring 3 days after infection and persisting indefinitely.

(ii) a high virus titre in the plasma (more than $10^8$ $ID_{50}$ per ml) 24 hours after infection with persistence of the viraemia at a lower level ($10^4$ $ID_{50}$ per ml) for the remainder of the animal's life.

The only other infectious agent which can cause a comparable alteration in plasma LDH activity without causing severe illness or death is *Eperythrozoon coccoides*, a murine pathogen frequently found in association with transplantable tumours (ARISON, CASSARO, and SHONK, 1963). The increase in plasma LDH activity caused by *Eperythrozoon coccoides* is usually less than that produced by LDV infection, but depends on the severity of the eperythrozoon infection. In splenectomized or tumour bearing animals, the parasitaemia is greater and more prolonged and the rise in plasma LDH activity higher that in intact mice. However, the LDH level always returns to normal, usually within 10 to 14 days (RILEY, LOVELESS, and FITZMAURICE, 1964). LDV and *Eperythrozoon coccoides* have a synergistic effect on the plasma LDH level in doubly infected mice. The parasitaemia and splenomegaly are also more severe in LDV infected animals (RILEY, 1964; STANSLY and NEILSON, 1965). The spleen appears to play a major role in limiting infection with *Eperythrozoon coccoides* and probably the impaired function of the reticuloendothelial system in LDV infected mice accounts for the more prolonged parasitaemia.

In any case of doubt as to the agent causing a rise in plasma LDH activity, the presence of *Eperythrozoon coccoides* should be excluded. Test material is injected into splenectomized mice and stained blood films examined by light microscopy 2, 4, 6, 8 and 10 days later for the bodies characteristic of *Eperythrozoon coccoides*. Alternatively, mice can be injected with 0.5 mg of oxophenarsine hydrochloride at the same time as the test material. Oxophenarsine hydrochloride has no effect on LDV infection and does not prevent the rise in plasma LDH activity but it prevents infection with *Eperythrozoon coccoides* and growth of the organism in animals already infected (ARISON, CASSARO, and SHONK, 1963; RILEY, LOVELESS, and FITZMAURICE, 1964).

It might reasonably be expected that any virus infection causing tissue damage would result in an elevated level of plasma enzyme activity (RILEY, HUERTO, BARDELL, FITZMAURICE, and LOVELESS, 1963). However, in a study of the plasma enzyme levels in mice infected with vaccinia virus, influenza virus A (strain PR8), lymphocytic choriomeningitis virus (LCM) and encephalomyocarditis virus (EMC), no changes were observed except with EMC virus (MAHY, ROWSON, SALAMAN, and PARR, 1964). When injected intramuscularly or intraperitoneally, EMC virus caused gross damage to muscular tissue and a rise in LDH activity in the plasma comparable to that produced by LDV, but EMC virus causes a rapidly lethal disease and so the two infections are not likely to be confused. Injected intracerebrally, EMC virus, like LCM virus, causes little change in plasma enzyme levels.

This suggests that cerebral damage releases little enzyme activity into the circulation. In addition to the increase in plasma LDH activity in EMC virus infected mice, there is an increase in plasma aldolase and aspartate transaminase activities, which are normal in LDV infected mice (Fig. 6).

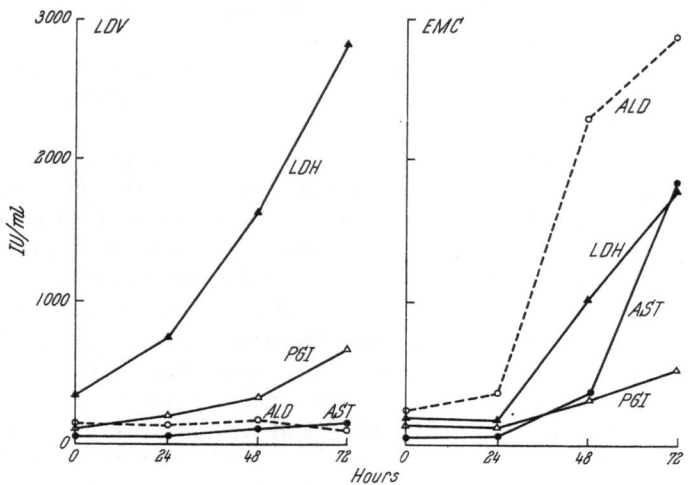

Fig. 6. Changes in plasma aldolase (ALD), aspartate transaminase (AST), lactic dehydrogenase (LDH) and phosphoglucose isomerase (PGI) activities in mice up to 72 hours after intraperitoneal injection with either LDV or encephalomyocarditis (EMC) virus. (From MAHY, ROWSON, SALAMAN, and PARR, 1964)

The failure of influenza A virus infection to cause a rise in plasma LDH activity is surprising as this virus causes an increased level of LDH activity in the chorioallantoic fluid of infected eggs (KELLY and GREIFF, 1961). Possibly the proportion of cells killed in the influenza virus-infected mouse is much less than in the infected egg, but a more likely explanation is that enzymes released from damaged cells accumulate in the egg, whereas in the mouse, most of the damaged cell contents are released into the respiratory passages and are not absorbed into the circulation.

Ectromelia virus causes a raised plasma LDH level associated with damage to the liver and cardiac muscle (GEORGII, 1964). Newcastle disease virus has been reported to cause a raised plasma LDH level twelve days after infection (WENNER, MILLIAN, MIRAND, and GRACE, 1962). However, many virus preparations are contaminated with LDV and the authors of this report do not give the source of the Newcastle disease virus or any details which would indicate whether the rise in plasma LDH activity was due to Newcastle disease or a mixed infection.

The mouse leukaemia viruses are frequently found to be contaminated with LDV but this is not because these viruses have any biological interdependence. It results from the fact that many leukaemia viruses are maintained by frequent animal passage and several of them were isolated from mice bearing tumours which were already infected with LDV. When free of LDV, the mouse leukaemia viruses and polyoma virus have no effect on plasma LDH activity before the neoplastic process is well advanced (MAHY, ROWSON, SALAMAN, and PARR, 1964). Other viruses such as LCM virus (GLEDHILL and ROWSON, 1965), scrapie virus

(ADAMS and FIELD, 1967) and mouse hepatitis virus (NOTKINS, BERRY, MOLONEY, and GREENFIELD, 1962) have been found to be mixed with LDV. *Eperythrozoon coccoides* has also been found contaminated with LDV (RILEY, LOVELESS, and FITZMAURICE, 1964).

The separation of LDV from other viruses is relatively easy by end-point dilution. Few if any viruses will produce a level of viraemia 24 hours after infection comparable with that in LDV infected mice. If the plasma of mice 24 hours after infection is serially diluted to $10^{-11}$ and the higher dilutions injected into pathogen-free mice, a pure LDV infection will be obtained in most cases. Alternatively, LDV can be freed from larger viruses by filtration through a filter of average pore diameter 80 nm.

The purification and concentration of LDV by centrifugation is possible providing this is done at low temperature (NOTKINS and SHOCAT, 1963). DU BUY and JOHNSON (1965) diluted their crude virus preparation with an equal volume of 0.3 M potassium citrate and 0.003 per cent hyaluronidase and digested at room temperature for one hour before differential centrifugation and resuspension of the virus pellet in one-tenth the original volume of distilled water. They further purified the virus by petroleum ether extraction which resulted in the loss of one to two logs of infectivity.

A number of workers have been unable to deposit all the infectivity in LDV preparations by centrifugation and have postulated that two particles are present (ADAMS and BOWMAN, 1964; STARK and CRISPENS, 1965). There is no supporting evidence for the presence of two different types of virus particle but there is evidence that some of the virus is combined with antibodies which do not cause inactivation of infectivity and these particles may have somewhat different physical properties (see p. 78).

The only method available for titrating LDV is to inoculate serial dilutions into groups of mice and to measure their plasma LDH activity after 3 days to determine which mice have been infected. The method is easy but requires a large amount of animal space and laboratory time. However, the work involved in the large number of LDH estimations can be reduced by two methods. DU BUY and JOHNSON (1965) pooled measured blood samples from the mice in a group and performed one LDH determination on the pooled plasma. From a Table constructed experimentally, they were able to estimate the number of infected mice in the group from the LDH activity of the pooled serum. This method proved satisfactory in their hands but is not aesthetically very satisfying. Another method described by ROWSON, MAHY, and SALAMAN (1965) is to perform a qualitative colorimetric test on individual sera using a modification of the method originally described by KELLY and GREIFF (1961). The difference in plasma LDH activity between the normal and infected mice is so great that a single spot test performed in a depression plate will reliably indicate infection (Fig. 7). This method has the advantage of giving results on individual mice and is much less laborious than quantitative estimations.

Other methods of virus titration such as haemagglutination and growth in tissue culture have been attempted. CRISPENS (1965a) found no agglutination of chicken, sheep, rabbit, guinea pig or human group 0 erythrocytes at 4° or 25° C by LDV. Most workers who have grown LDV in tissue cultures have been unable to observe any morphological alteration in the cells or increase in LDH activity

in the medium (see p. 63). FRANTSI and GREGORY (1969) have reported a cytopathogenic effect and an increase in LDH activity in the medium of LDV infected
cells. The cytopathogenic effect was reproducible with difficulty and it would
seem that, unless the method of obtaining sensitive cells can be improved, the test
would not be suitable for titration of virus preparations. The haemagglutination
negative plaque test described by CARVER, MARCUS, and SETO (1967) in which

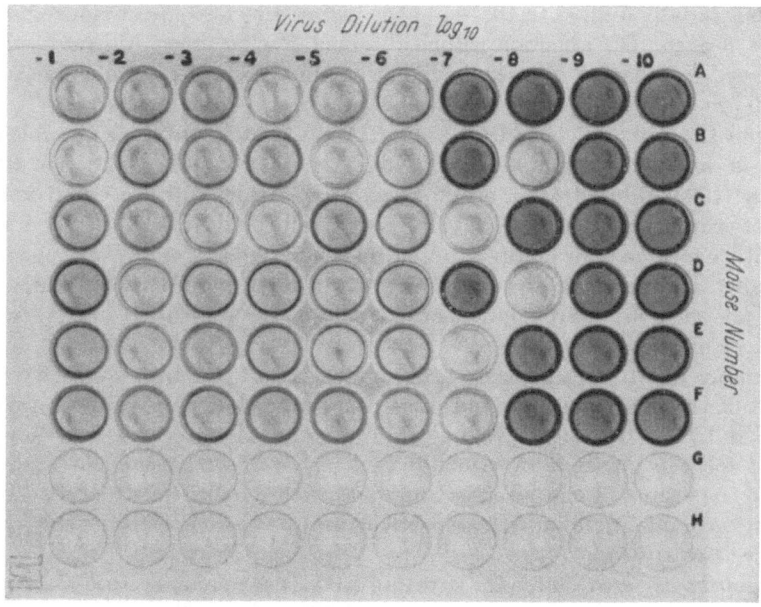

Fig. 7. Photograph of haemagglutination tray used for qualitative plasma LDH tests in a titration of LDV.
Each well contains the plasma from one mouse and six mice were used at each 10-fold dilution. The dark wells
indicate low LDH activity and absence of LDV infection

confluent haemadsorption to Newcastle disease virus-infected cells is specifically
inhibited by a number of different viruses was reported to work as a plaque test
for LDV (MARCUS and CARVER, 1967 and 1969). The test is satisfactory if mouse
embryo tissue cultures can be obtained which will support the growth of Newcastle
disease virus but cultures are very unreliable in this respect and CARVER (1969)
has not found the test satisfactory for LDV. The reason why mouse embryo tissue
cultures are so variable in their response to Newcastle disease virus may be that
they contain interfering viruses.

# IV. Properties of the Virus

## A. Morphology

The morphological appearance of a virus in the electron microscope is frequently
one of the simplest criteria to be established in classification, and serological relationships will probably be found to exist only between viruses which are morpho-

logically similar (ALMEIDA and WATERSON, 1969). Identification of viruses under the electron microscope usually relies on the observation of large populations of similar looking particles showing a characteristic fine structure (DE HARVEN, 1965), but despite the fact that high titres of infectious LDV can be detected in the plasma of infected mice 24 hours after infection (see p. 43), early attempts to demonstrate the agent by electron microscopy of the pellet deposited from plasma at $100,000 \times g$ failed to reveal any particles which were not also present in a pellet from uninfected mouse plasma (ROWSON and HORNE, 1962). However, in 1963 BLADEN and NOTKINS published electron micrographs of plasma pellets, negatively stained with phosphotungstic acid (PTA), showing essentially spheroidal particles $69 \, nm \times 76 \, nm$ in diameter. These particles were not found in similarly prepared plasma pellets from either uninfected mice, or mice which had received ether-inactivated virus 24 hours earlier (BLADEN and NOTKINS, 1963). Plasma from mice infected with LDV for 9 days contained less than one particle per electron microscope field, although the virus titre in the plasma at this time is around $10^7 \, ID_{50}/ml$ plasma (NOTKINS, 1965 a). One explanation for this might be that the particle to infectivity ratio is very low indeed, approaching that of bacterial viruses (LURIA, WILLIAMS, and BACKUS, 1951). Particle to infectivity ratios for most animal viruses are at least 10 and may be as high as $10^7$ (ISAACS, 1957).

The particles thought to be LDV in these early electron micrographs showed little evidence of fine structure, although it was reported that in addition to the spheroidal particles some 'tailed' forms were present, similar to those observed with the mouse leukaemia viruses (DALTON, HAGUENAU, and MOLONEY, 1962; ZEIGEL and RAUSCHER, 1963). Since the tailed forms were rarely seen in plasma pellets which had been fixed in osmium tetroxide prior to negative staining (BLADEN and NOTKINS, 1963), it was concluded that they were artifacts produced in the preparation and staining of the virus.

In 1964, CRISPENS and BURNS reported a morphological study of LDV by thin-sectioning of plasma pellets derived from infected and uninfected mice. A pellet prepared from infected mice (infectivity titre, $10^{10} \, ID_{50}/ml$) was fixed in 1 per cent osmic acid with veronal buffer, pH 7.4, dehydrated and embedded in methacrylate. Thin sections cut from this material and stained in lead citrate revealed oval-shaped particles, 15 nm wide by 45 nm long; the latter measurement is identical to the diameter of LDV as calculated from Gradocol filtration studies (ROWSON, MAHY, and SALAMAN, 1963). These oval particles were not present in plasma pellets prepared from uninfected mice or in a 100 nm average pore diameter Millipore filtrate of a human breast carcinoma. It was suggested (CRISPENS and BURNS, 1964) that the differences in particle shape and size between this and the previous study by BLADEN and NOTKINS (1963) resulted from the use of thin-sectioning as opposed to negative-staining techniques.

DE THÉ and NOTKINS (1965) reached a similar conclusion. Osmium-fixed pellets prepared from viraemic plasma and examined in thin section revealed oval or elliptical particles 36—42 nm wide and 45—75 nm long, as well as some rounded particles 40 nm in diameter which were thought to be cross sections of the elliptical ones (Fig. 8a). However, negatively-stained pellets of unfixed material contained larger and more pleomorphic particles, 60—65 nm in diameter by 70—85 nm in length, including 'tailed' forms (DE THÉ and NOTKINS, 1965). It was concluded

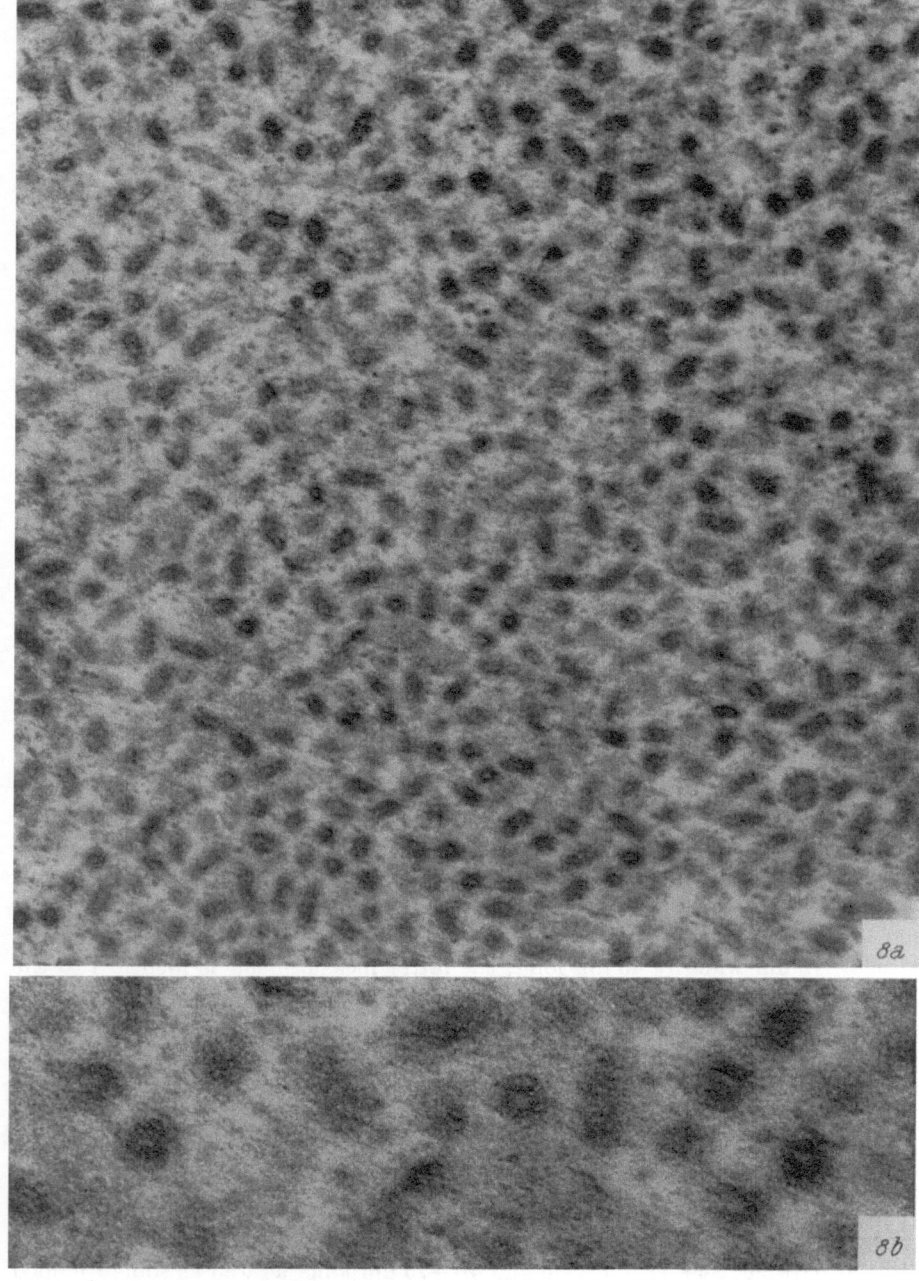

Fig. 8. Thin section of an osmium-fixed pellet prepared from viraemic mouse plasma.

a) Elliptical or oblong particles 36—42 nm wide and 45—75 nm long, and rounded particles averaging 40 nm in
diameter are present. Magnification ×125,000

b) Higher magnification showing nucleoids 26—29 nm in diameter surrounded by a thin envelope separated from
the nucleoid by an electron lucent space 5 to 7 nm wide. Magnification ×310,000 (From DE THÉ and NOTKINS, 1965)

that the negative-staining technique used was introducing artifacts into the preparation. Similar aberrant forms have been seen in preparations of murine leukaemia viruses, and these are probably caused by the transient hypertonicity which occurs during the desiccation of the viruses on the electron microscope grid, because of salts present in the suspension medium and in phosphotungstic acid solutions (LEVY, BOIRON, SILVESTRE, and BERNARD, 1965).

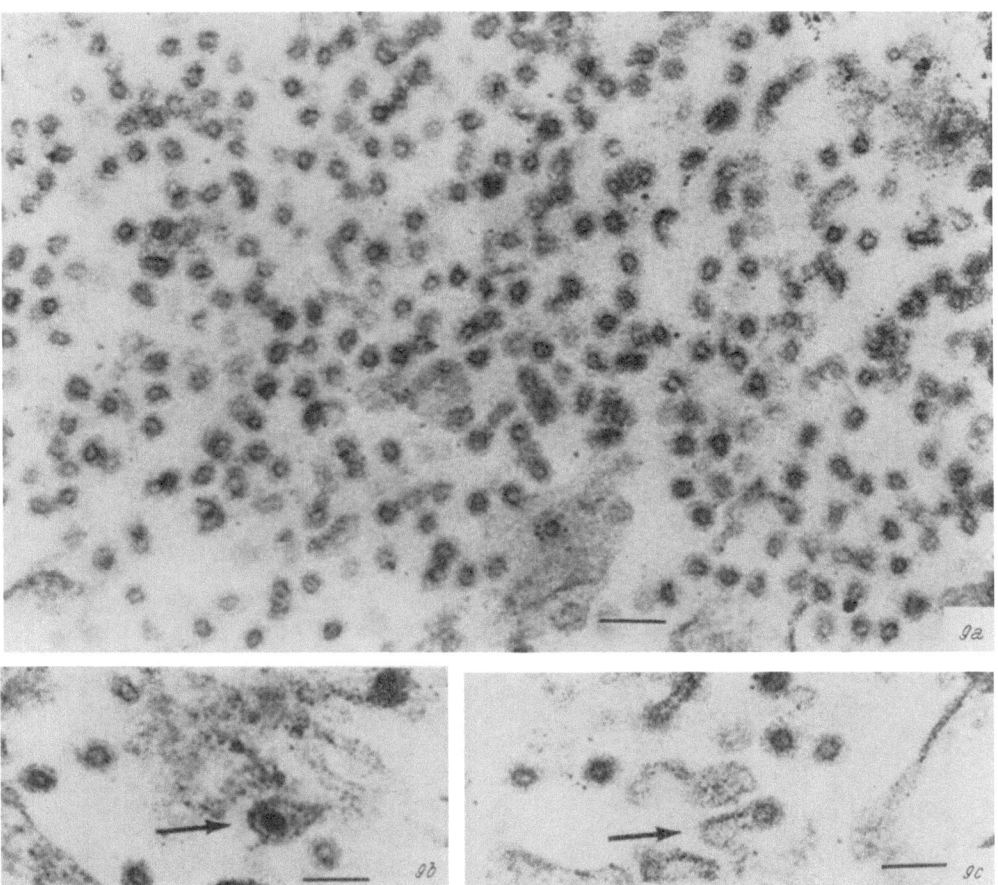

Fig. 9. Thin sections of osmium-fixed plasma pellets.
a) Characteristic particles showing inner and outer rings
b) and c) Selected areas each showing a single membrane bound particle. The lines represent 100 nm. (From DU BUY and JOHNSON, 1965)

Results consistent with those of CRISPENS and BURNS (1964) and DE THÉ and NOTKINS (1965) were reported by RILEY (1968b). He observed closely-packed particles having a mean diameter of 35 to 40 nm in thin sections of viraemic plasma pellets. No such particles were found in any of 280 separate sections of a normal plasma pellet which were examined.

Observations on the structure of LDV were made by DE HARVEN and FRIEND (1966), quite by chance during a study of the ultrastructure of Friend virus. Since

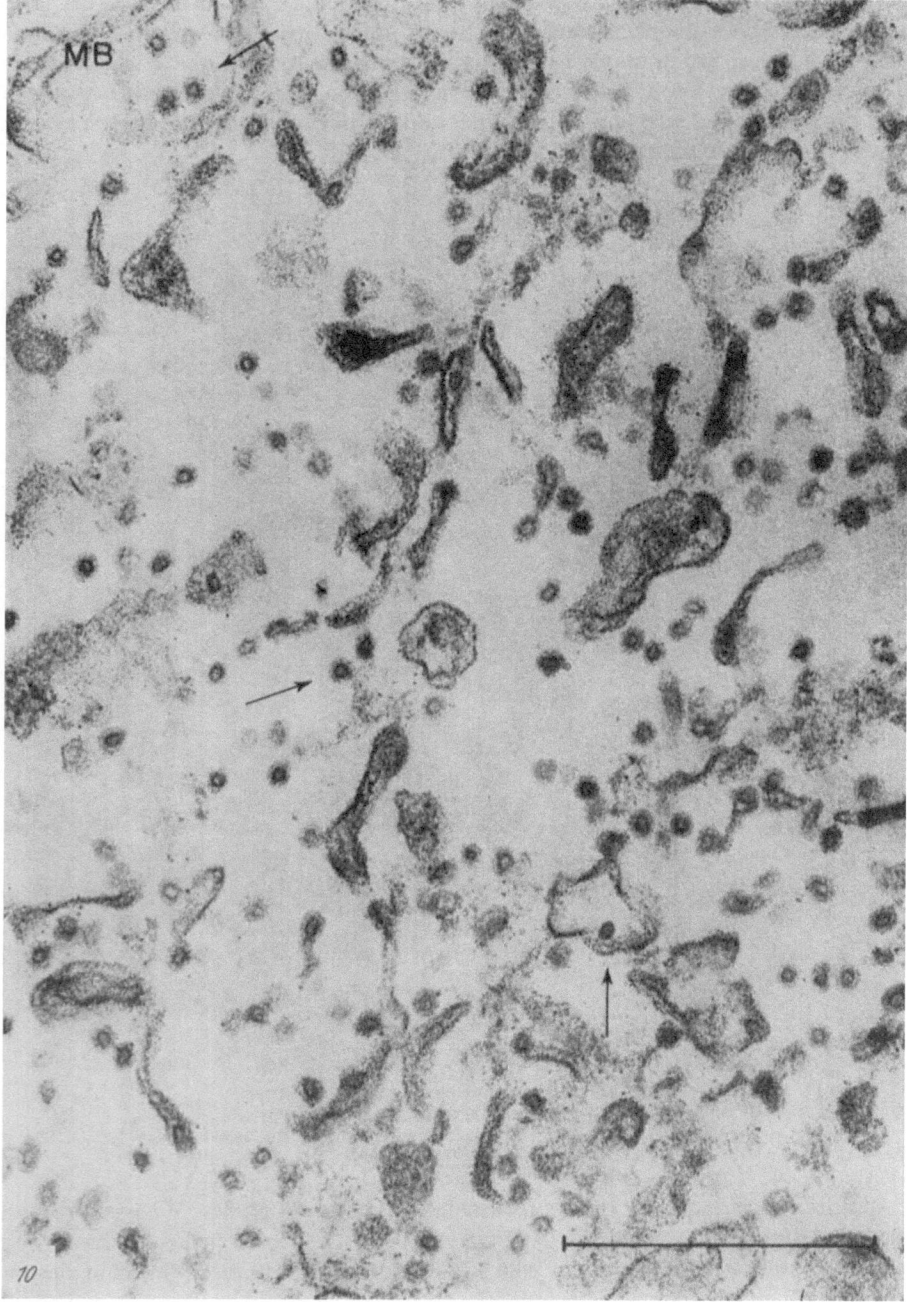

Fig. 10. Section of a pellet of partially purified virus obtained from Ehrlich tumour ascites fluid.
The LDV consists of a dense inner annulus of 25 nm diameter and a less distinct outer halo of 50 nm diameter
(arrows). One or more of these particles may be bounded by an additional membrane (MB). The bar represents
500 nm. (From Du Buy and Johnson, 1966)

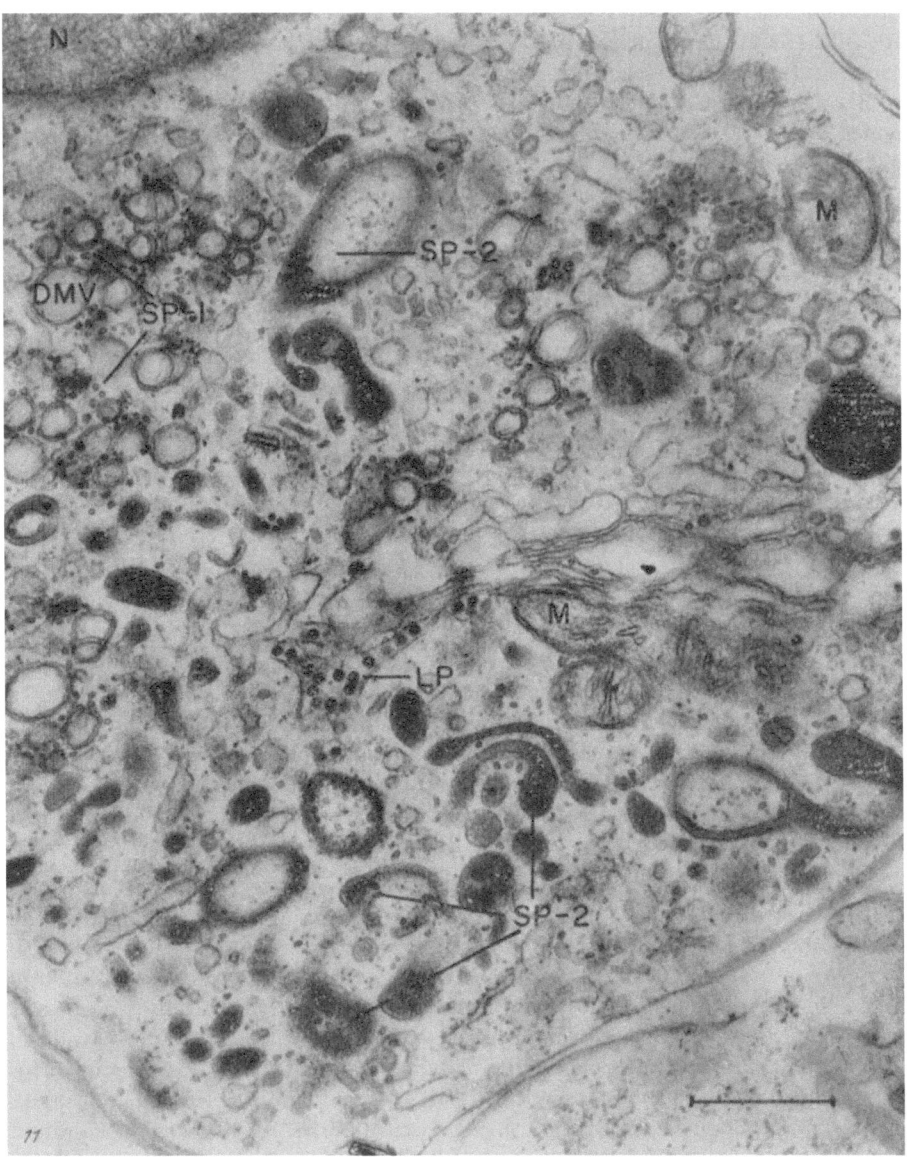

Fig. 11. Section of lymph node cells, 24 hours after infection.
Small uniform annular particles of 25 nm diameter (SP-1) are seen scattered among double membraned vesicles (DMV) and occasionally within single membraned dense particles (SP-2). The larger particles (LP) of 50 nm diameter with a halo are usually associated in varying numbers with irregular single membranes. Apparently normal mitochondria (M) and part of the nucleus (N) are identified. The bar represents 500 nm. (From Du Buy and Johnson, 1966)

the stock of Friend virus which they used was contaminated with LDV, high-speed pellets obtained from filtered plasma of DBA/2 mice at 24 hours after virus inoculation contained large numbers of LDV particles. These were easily distinguishable because of their smaller size from the 100 nm diameter Friend leukaemia virus particles which appeared in the plasma at 3 to 4 days after inoculation. The particles assumed to be LDV measured approximately half the size of leukaemia virus particles, and were of two different types. Most of the particles were oblong, 70 nm long by 35 nm wide, with an indistinct envelope and an electron-lucent core in the centre. The other particles appeared spherical, 57 nm in diameter, and with a small electron-dense doughnut-shaped core, 25 to 28 nm in diameter. In some cases, all the particles appeared spherical which would not support the idea that the spherical particles were cross-sections of the oblong ones.

Spherical particles of similar morphology were observed by DU BUY and JOHN-SON (1965, 1966) in virus preparations purified from ascites fluid obtained from mice bearing the Ehrlich ascites carcinoma (Fig. 9a). The typical particles consisted of a dense inner ring of about 25 nm diameter, and a less dense and sometimes indistinct outer ring extending to about 50 nm. Occasionally the particles were seen within single-membraned vesicles (Figs. 9b, 9c, 10). The presence of oblong or elliptical particles was not reported by DU BUY and JOHNSON (1965).

The detailed fine structural features of the spherical particles were described by DE THÉ and NOTKINS (1965). These particles contain a nucleoid, 26 to 29 nm in diameter, consisting of a dense shell 7 to 9 nm wide with an electron lucent inner core. Surrounding the dense shell of the nucleoid is an outer layer, 5 to 7 nm wide, of lower density, limited by a thin outer membrane (Fig. 8b). DE THÉ and NOTKINS (1965) also examined the liver, kidney, spleen, lymph nodes, thymus, bone marrow, lung, mammary gland, and peritoneal macrophages from infected mice for the presence of similar particles. None was found except in a small percentage of the peritoneal macrophages, where they occurred in close association with the cell surface and with the membrane of and within cytoplasmic vacuoles.

The presence of LDV particles in macrophages from infected mice was confirmed by DU BUY and JOHNSON (1966), who examined lymph nodes and spleens at various stages of infection up to 24 hours. The characteristic spherical particles, 50 nm diameter and containing a nucleoid of 25 nm diameter, were found in large numbers in the cytoplasm of certain lymph nodes (never in the nuclei), and in germinal centre cells of the spleen (Figs. 11—14). In addition, they observed the nucleoid alone, as a 25 nm dense annulus; they concluded that this nucleoid was a developmental form of the mature LDV particle. It is interesting that no naked nucleoids were observed by DE THÉ and NOTKINS (1965) who however examined peritoneal macrophages rather than lymph node cells. A more detailed ultra-structural study of LDV in mouse lymphoid tissue was made by SNODGRASS and HANNA (1970) who observed the virus particles in close intercellular association with phagocytic reticular cells in splenic lymphoid nodules (Figs. 15—17). The particles consisted of a dark nucleoid, 25 nm in diameter, with an electron lucent core, and an outer electron lucent envelope measuring 45 to 50 nm in total diameter. The presence of oblong or elliptical particles was not reported, and no small naked nucleoids were detected even in the cytoplasm. Virus particles were frequently

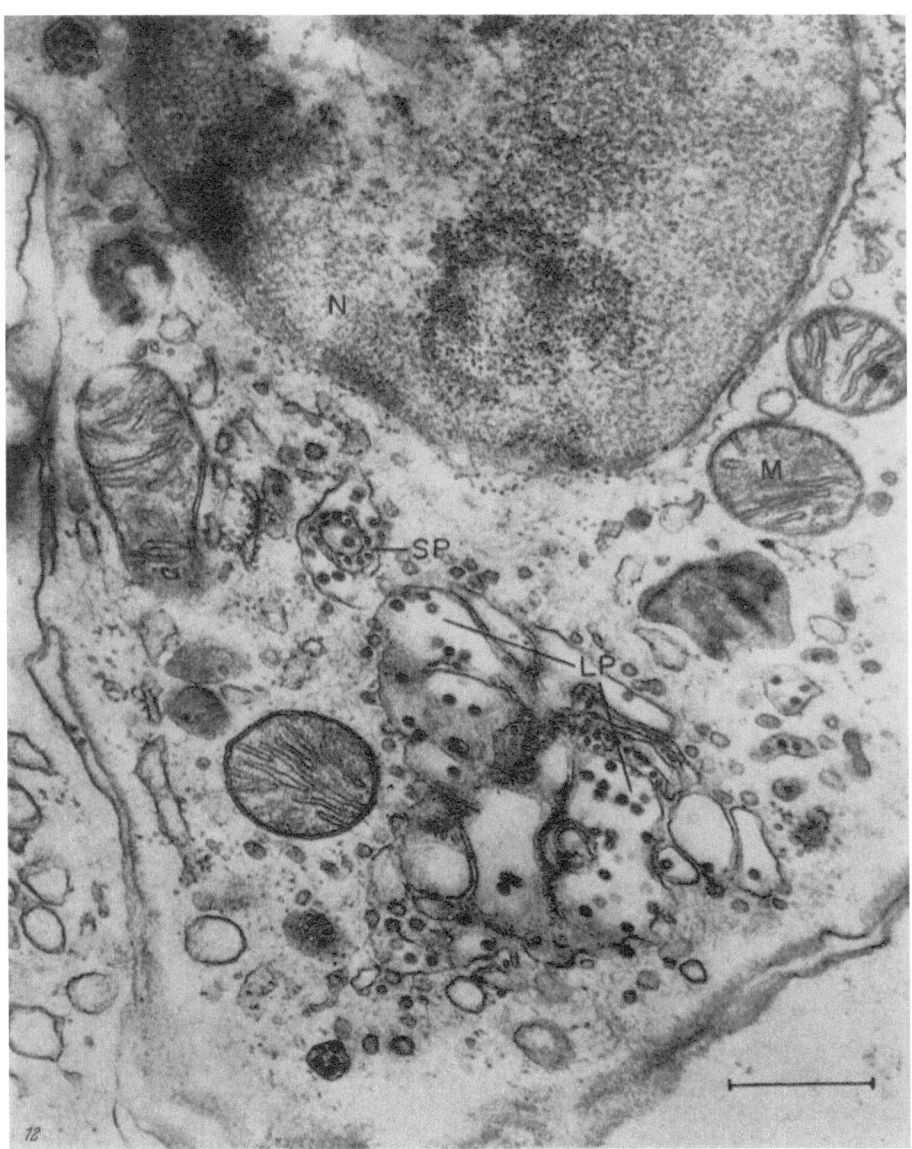

Fig. 12. Section of lymph node cell, 24 hours after infection.
Small and large particles can be seen, associated with single membraned vesicles. (M) mitochondria; (N) nucleus; (SP) small particles; (LP) large particles. The bar represents 500 nm. (From Du Buy and Johnson, 1966)

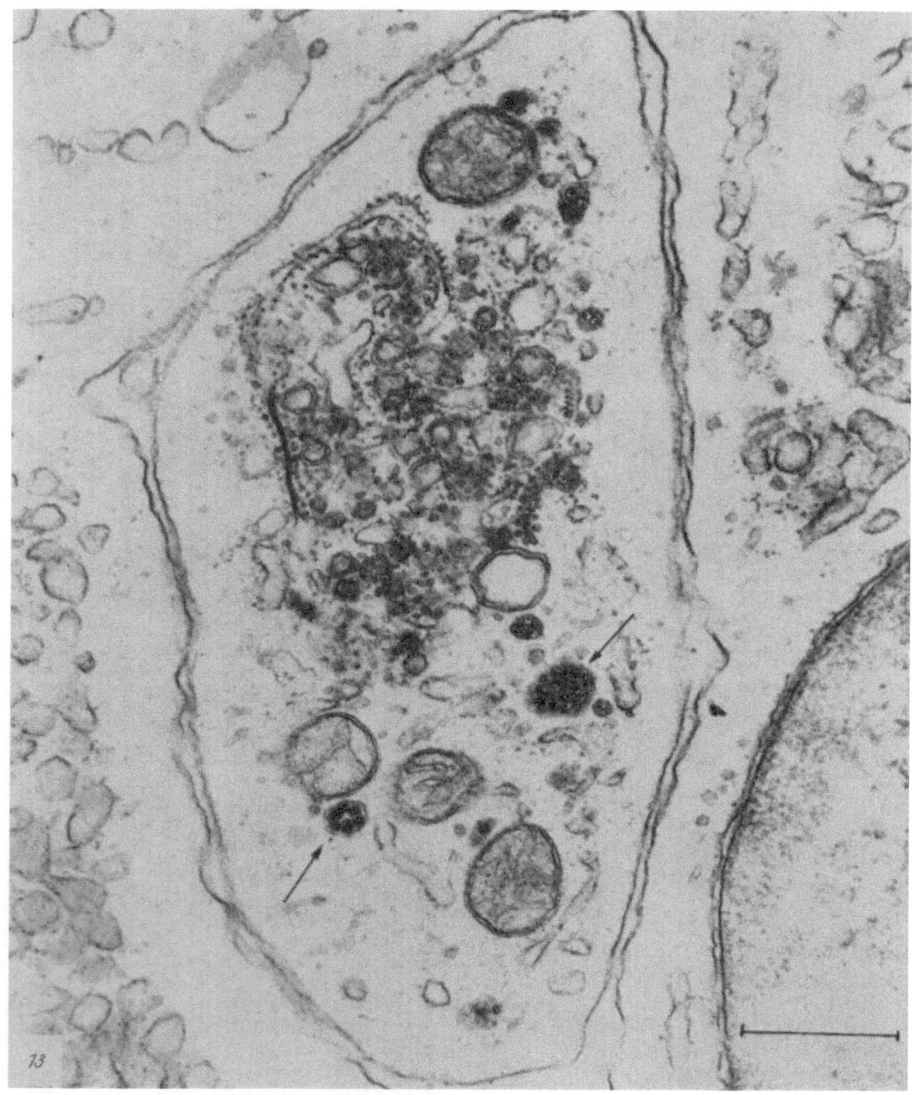

Fig. 13. Section of lymph cell, 24 hours after infection.
Small particles and intravesicular aggregates (arrows) predominate. The bar represents 500 nm. (From Du Buy and Johnson, 1966)

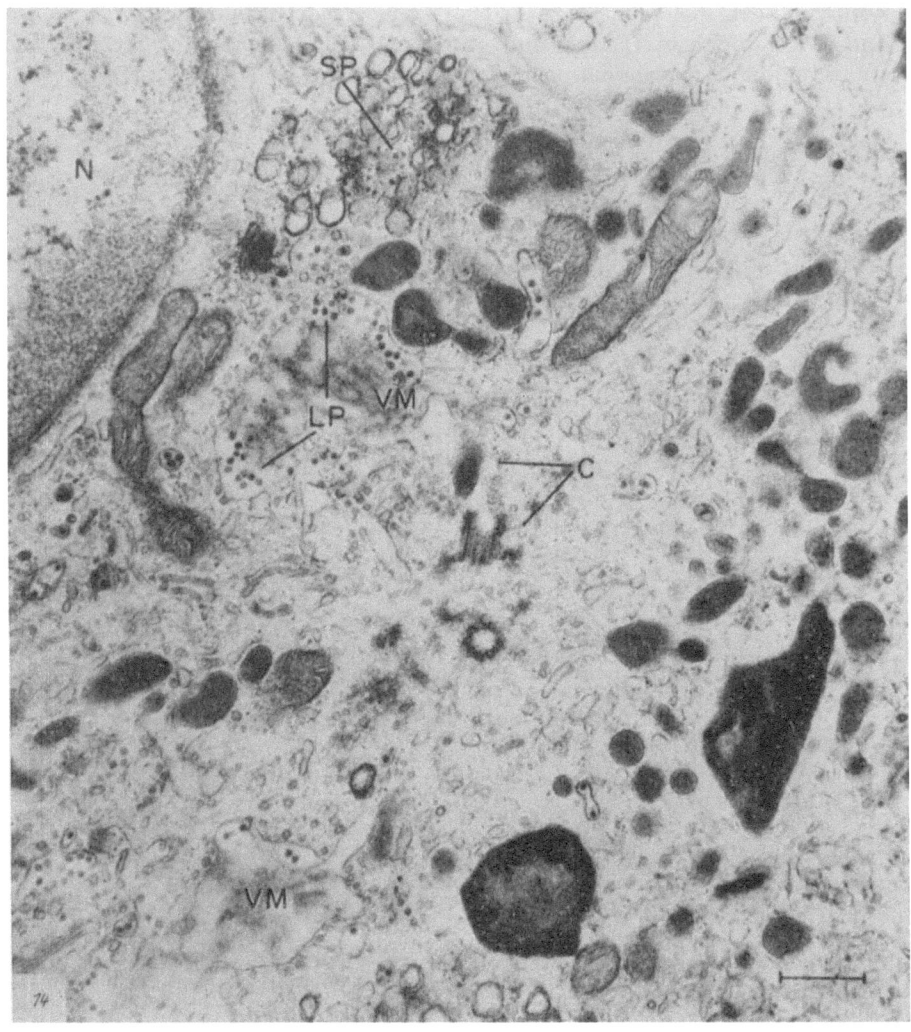

Fig. 14. Lymph node cells 18 hours after infection.
There are many small extra-vesicular particles (SP) and large intravesicular particles (LP). It is possible that the halo is derived from some of the vesicular material (VM). Just to the lower right of centre a pair of centrioles (C) is visible, (N) nucleus. The bar represents 500 nm. (From Du Buy and Johnson, 1966)

aligned intercellularly in uniform rows, and a few were contained in single membrane-bound intracellular vesicles (Fig. 15).

With the development of a method for *in vitro* cultivation of LDV in mouse
peritoneal macrophages (EVANS and SALAMAN, 1965), another source of virus
became available for examination by electron microscopy (PROSSER and EVANS,

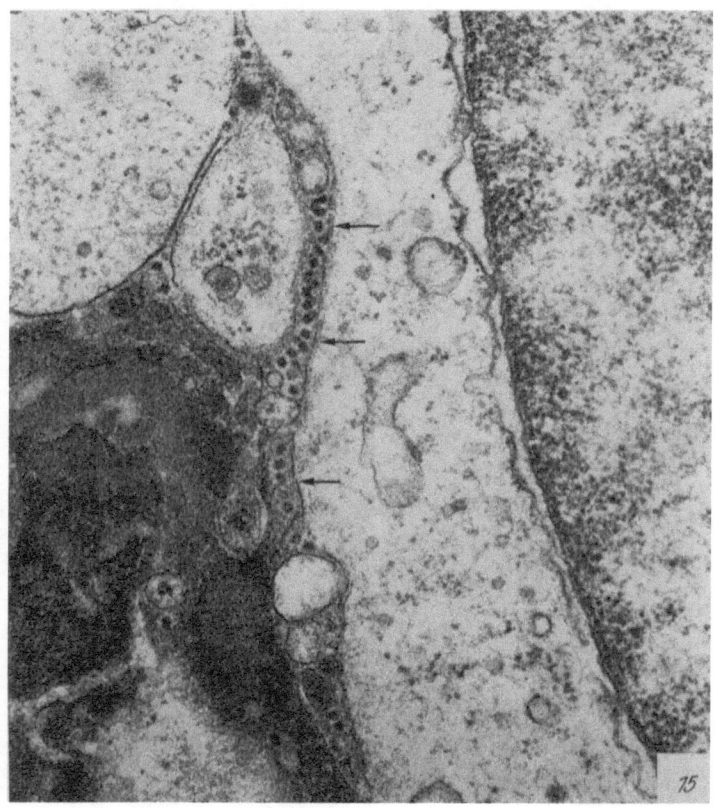

Fig. 15. Sections of thymic-dependent area of splenic lymphoid nodule.
LDV particles (arrows) with 25 nm diameter nucleoids and 45—50 nm diameter envelopes are localized intercellularly. Uranyl acetate and lead citrate. Magnification × 52,000. (From SNODGRASS and HANNA, 1970)

1967). Cells from several infected cultures were pooled, deposited by centrifugation, and the pellets fixed in osmium tetroxide before thin sectioning. Four different types of particle were observed in the infected cells, but two types predominated
(Figs. 18 and 19). These were large, round particles (type 1) with an average
external diameter of 51 nm, containing a dense nucleoid having an average diameter of 31 nm, and small round or oval particles (type 3), of similar appearance
to the nucleoid of the large particle, with an average external diameter of 33 nm
(Figs. 18 and 19). These two types of particle observed by PROSSER and EVANS
correspond closely with those in macrophages from infected mice by DU BUY
and JOHNSON (1966). In addition to these two predominant particles, large elongated (type 2) and small rod-shaped (type 4) forms were seen less frequently (PROSSER

and EVANS, 1967). The particles were usually enclosed, often in neat bundles, by a single membrane which was continuous with the endoplasmic reticulum. The bundles usually contained particles either of types 1 and 2 or of types 3 and 4. However, all four types of particle were occasionally seen in the same cell. The distribution of particles amongst the cells studied was of particular interest; most cells contained no virus particles, and cells in which virus was seen usually contained large numbers of particles and often showed cytopathic changes.

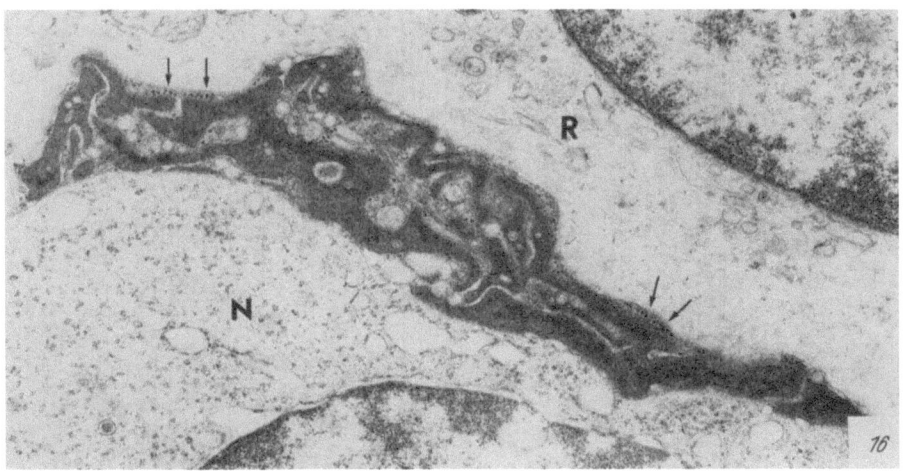

Fig. 16. Section of thymic-dependent area of splenic lymphoid nodule.
LDV particles (arrows) are apparently replicating from a phagocyte reticular cell (R) and migrating intercellularly between the processes of a dark reticular cell. Only one virus particle is seen between the dark reticular processes and the nonphagocytic cell (N) at bottom of field. Uranyl acetate and lead citrate. Magnification × 30,000. (From SNODGRASS and HANNA, 1970)

PROSSER and EVANS (1967) also examined pellets obtained from viraemic plasma, and found particles of similar dimensions and morphology to all four types seen in macrophage cultures. Elliptical forms, similar to those observed by previous workers (CRISPENS and BURNS, 1964; DE THÉ and NOTKINS, 1965; DE HARVEN and FRIEND, 1964) were frequently seen. These particles varied from 45 to 75 nm in length by 18 to 37 nm in width. Pellets prepared from the medium of infected macrophage cultures contained very few particles, presumably because of a much lower concentration of LDV than in plasma, but where seen the particles were of the same type as in plasma pellets. No similar particles were ever observed in control cultures, medium, or plasma (PROSSER and EVANS, 1967). Recently, DARNELL and PLAGEMANN (personal communication, 1974) have examined thin sections of plasma pellets from mice infected with LDV for 24 hours (Fig. 19a). They also found roughly spherical and elliptical particles, 40 to 50 nm in width by up to 70 nm in length. The particles, which were not found in uninfected mouse plasma, were characterized by an electron-dense nucleoid of 25 to 30 nm diameter and an outer double membrane (Fig. 19a). Of the four types of particle seen by them, PROSSER and EVANS favoured the large spherical particle (type 1), 51 nm in diameter, as being the mature, infective virion of LDV. This would be compatible with most size estimations by other criteria such as Gradocol membrane filtration (ROWSON *et al.*, 1963) or centrifugation data (RILEY, 1968 b). Also, a spherical particle of this size has been observed in the majority of electron microscopic investigations of LDV carried out so far (Table 3). A small spherical particle, observed by some workers, presumably represents the naked nucleoid of the mature virion. The role of the elliptical particles is not clear at present, but they might represent another virus associated with

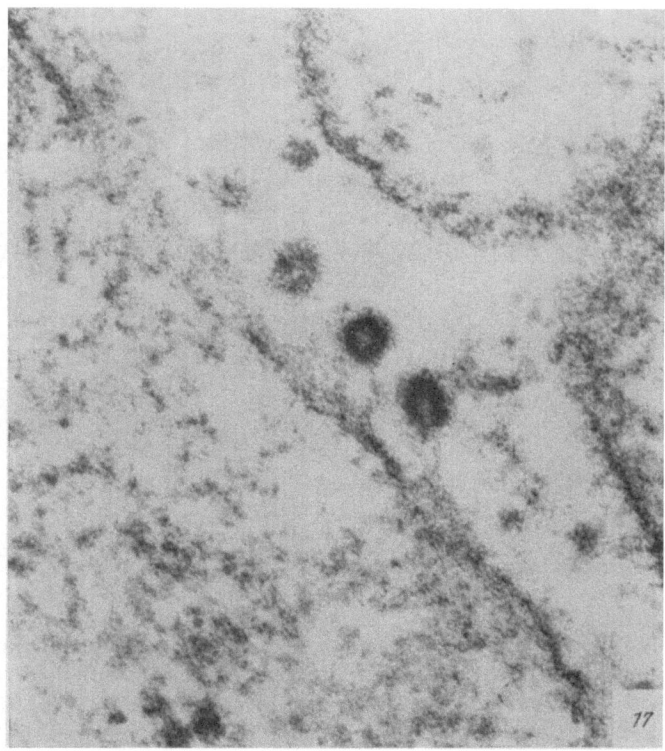

Fig. 17. Section of marginal zone of spleen.
Four virus particles can be seen cut at various levels. One at the right appears to be budding. The particles lie intercellularly and have filamentous attachments with the plasmalemma of a phagocytic reticular cell. The plasmalemma beneath the particles appears altered. Magnification × 210,000. (From SNODGRASS, LOWREY, and HANNA, 1972)

the LDV preparation. This could explain why they have only been seen by some investigators, as the preparations of LDV used by different workers clearly vary considerably in origin. Now that LDV can be cultivated in a number of different *in vitro* systems, it should be possible to make more accurate quantitative studies of the type of particle associated with LDV infectivity.

ALMEIDA and MIMS (1974) have applied the technique of immuno-electron microscopy (ALMEIDA and WATERSON, 1969) to the study of LDV. Using this technique on mouse plasma obtained from mice 18—24 hours after infection, they obtained pictures of large aggregates of virus-like particles (Fig. 20). The particles were bottle-shaped, each consisting of an elongated body and a less dense

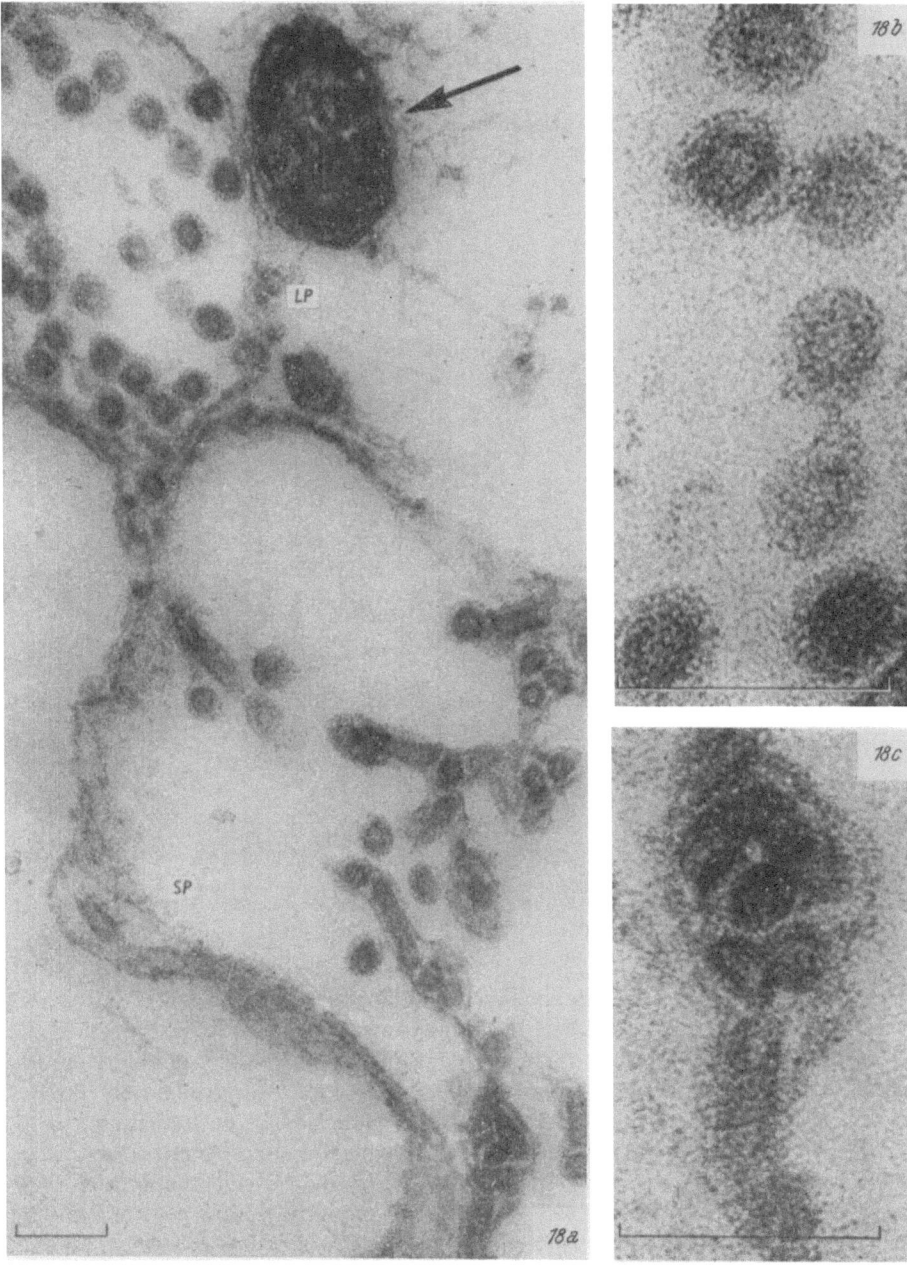

Fig. 18. Thin sections of peritoneal macrophage infected with LDV *in vitro*.
a) A bundle of large round particles, type 1 (LP). Rod-shaped, type 4 and small particles type 3 (SP) enveloped
closely by a membrane. A group of particles (indicated by arrow) is embedded in a dense amorphous substance
b) Photographic enlargement of large particles, type 1
c) Photographic enlargement of small and rod-shaped particles closely enveloped by a membrane. The lines
represent 100 nm. (From PROSSER and EVANS, 1967)

neck, with overall dimensions of 80—110 nm by 37—44 nm. The dense and more
uniform body was 65—73 nm by 37—44 nm. The neck could be as narrow as
14.5 nm but ranged in size up to the full width of the body of the particle, and
in some instances was even wider. Since the virus could only be found in reasonable
amounts after the addition of antiserum, it was difficult to obtain good resolution
on the surface of the particle. However, from the distribution of the antibody it

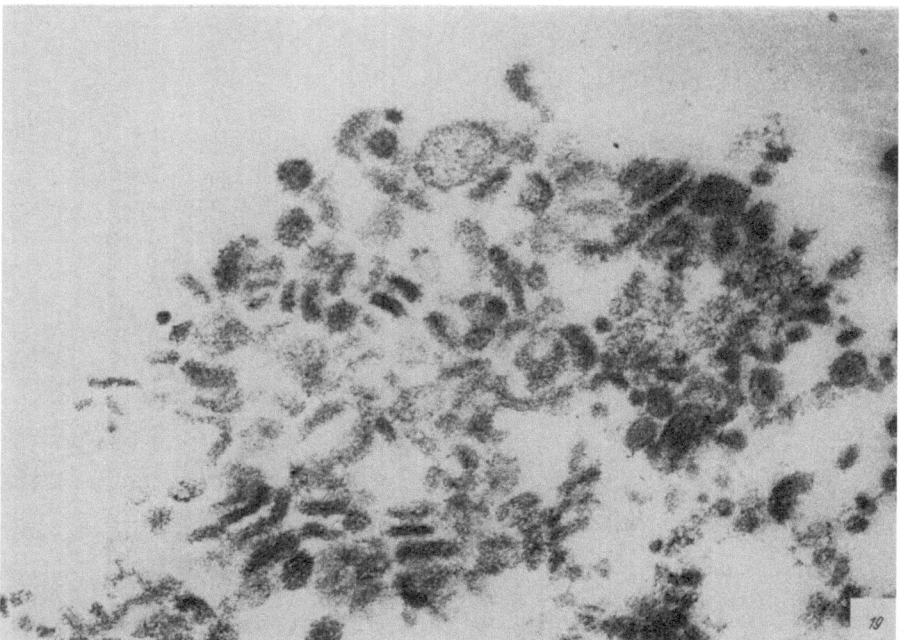

Fig. 19. Electron micrograph showing small rod-shaped particles type 4 in thin section of a pellet of partially
purified virus preparation from plasma of LDV infected mice. (From PROSSER and EVANS, 1967). Magnification
× 112.500

appeared that the particles might have a small surrounding fringe of projections.
The bottle-shaped particles were only found in fresh plasma. In plasma held at
4° C for 24 hours or stored for one week at —20°C the complexes consisted almost
entirely of pleomorphic but basically spherical particles approximately 60 by
90 nm. The bottle-shaped morphology of LDV particles can be interpreted as a
virus body 40 by 70 nm with a neck formed by the surrounding membrane that
could have been gained as the virus budded through the cell membrane. This
morphology of a virus particle with a membrane extending from it at one end is
seen with vesicular stomatitis virus and Bittner virus particles. The morphology
described by ALMEIDA and MIMS is in agreement with the appearances seen in thin
sections (Figs. 8 and 9), whereas in some of the earlier negatively stained preparations pleomorphic particles considerably larger than would be compatible with the
dimensions of the particles seen in sections were described. The importance of
using freshly harvested virus for studies of LDV morphology must not be forgotten.

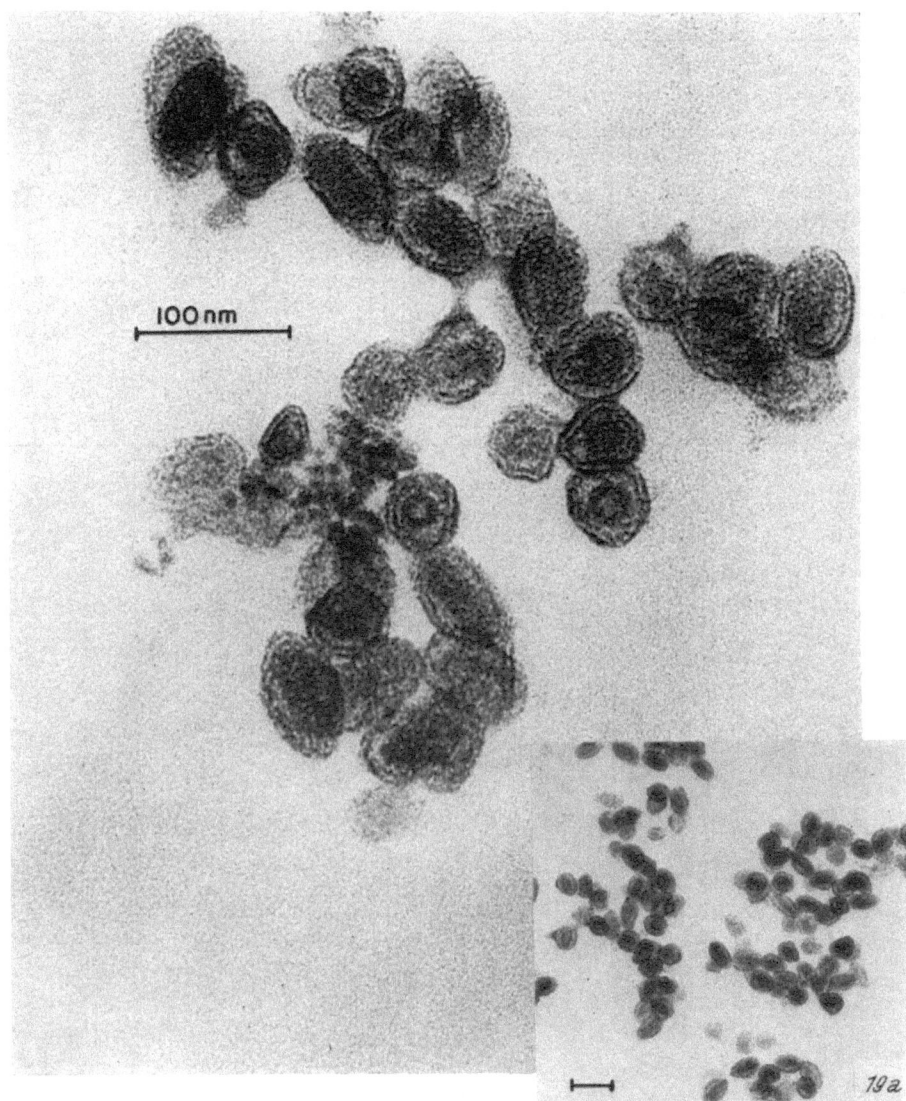

Fig. 19 a. Plasma obtained from mice infected for 24 hours with LDV, concentrated 30-fold by centrifugation (39,000 r. p. m. for 2.5 hours), repelleted, embedded, sectioned and stained with uranyl acetate. Photograph kindly supplied by Dr. P. G. W. PLAGEMANN

Table 3. *Reported Sizes of Particles Associated*

| Source | Large spherical | | Small spherical |
|---|---|---|---|
| | overall | core | |
| Plasma pellets | 70 | — | |
| Plasma pellets | | | |
| Plasma pellets and peritoneal macrophages | 40 | 26—29 | |
| Plasma pellets | 57 | 25—28 | |
| Plasma pellets | 50 | 25 | |
| Lymph Nodes | 50 | 25 | 25 |
| Peritoneal macrophages | 51 | 31 | 33 |
| Plasma pellets | 44 | 31 | 33 |
| Plasma pellets | 40 | | |
| Spleen | 45—50 | | 25 |
| Plasma antibody aggregates | After storage 60 × 90 | | |

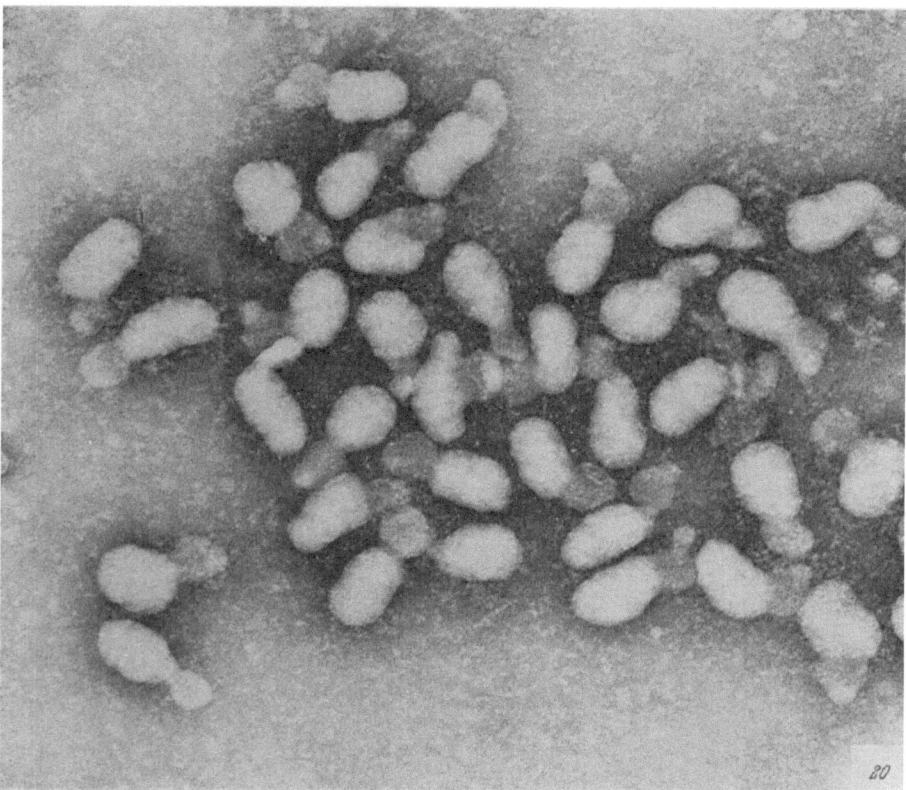

Fig. 20. A negatively stained clump of virus particles.

The virus and antibody were mixed and allowed to react overnight at 4° C. The virus antibody clumps were deposited by centrifugation at 15,000 r.p.m. for 1 hour, the deposit washed and negatively stained with 3 per cent phosphotungstic acid (pH 6) after resuspending in distilled water. Photograph kindly supplied by Dr. J. D. ALMEIDA *with Lactic Dehydrogenase Virus Infection (nm)*

| Elliptical | Other | Authors |
|---|---|---|
| | 'Tailed' forms | BLADEN and NOTKINS, 1963 |
| $15 \times 45$ | | CRISPENS and BURNS, 1964 |
| $36—42 \times 45—75$ | | DE THE and NOTKINS, 1965 |
| $35 \times 70$ | | DE HAVEN and FRIEND, 1966 |
| | | DU BUY and JOHNSON, 1965 |
| | | DU BUY and JOHNSON, 1966 |
| $20—38 \times 64—124$ | Large elongated forms | PROSSER and EVANS, 1967 |
| $18—37 \times 45—75$ | | PROSSER and EVANS, 1967 |
| | | RILEY, 1968 b |
| | | SNODGRASS and HANNA, 1970 |
| Fresh virus | "Bottle shaped" | ALMEIDA and MIMS, 1974 |
| $80—110 \times 37—44$ overall | particles | |
| $65—73 \times 37—44$ dense body | | |

## B. Physico-Chemical Structure

The diameter of the LDV virion has been determined by Gradocol membrane filtration and found to be 45 to 55 nm (NOTKINS and SHOCHAT, 1963; ROWSON, MAHY, and SALAMAN, 1963; DU BUY and JOHNSON, 1965). The estimate of 45 nm (ROWSON, MAHY, and SALAMAN, 1963) was based on the finding that viral infectivity just passed a membrane of average pore diameter 74 nm and was held back by a membrane of 67 nm. The earlier size estimations by RILEY (1963 a), in which a size of 2 nm was concluded to be the diameter of the infectious particle have not been confirmed and appear to have been erroneous (ROWSON, MAHY, and SALAMAN, 1963; DU BUY and JOHNSON, 1965). Nevertheless, perhaps as a result of RILEY's suggestion that the virus was in reality a 'minute infectious entity' (RILEY 1963 a), several workers have investigated the possibility that preparations of LDV contain, in addition to the 45 nm particle, a smaller infectious particle of different physical properties. Thus, both CRISPENS (1964 c) and ADAMS and BOWMAN (1964) found that ultracentrifugation of plasma obtained from mice which had been infected for 24 hours resulted in a reduction of supernatant infectious titre from $10^{11}$ to $10^7$ $ID_{50}$ per ml, and suggested that the residual infectivity which did not sediment after 4 hours at $105,000 \times g$ represented a 'small particle'. RILEY, CAMPBELL, LOVELESS, and FITZMAURICE (1964) and RILEY (1968 b) reached a similar conclusion, based on the sedimentation properties of LDV in density gradients prepared using the density gradient trap method of POLSON and VAN REGENMORTEL (1961). As a reference virus, Rous sarcoma virus was employed. Under conditions of centrifugation (30,000 r.p.m. in a Spinco SW39L rotor for 10 minutes) in which Rous sarcoma virus was completely sedimented beyond the 1 cm sampling point, a considerable level of LDV infectivity remained in the supernatant. After 30 minutes centrifugation, there was a decrease of titre from $10^9$ to $10^4$ $ID_{50}$/ml, but longer periods of centrifugation up to 2 hours did not reduce this titre any further (Fig. 21). Since the gradient trap method is designed to prevent virus contamination of the supernatant by convection or stir-back (POLSON and VAN REGENMORTEL, 1961) RILEY concluded that the plateau of infectivity reached after 30 minutes was due to the presence of a particle of either low density or small size. The virus which did sediment within 30 minutes ('large particle') was calculated to have an $S_{20, w}$ value of 150 to 175, and a mean particle

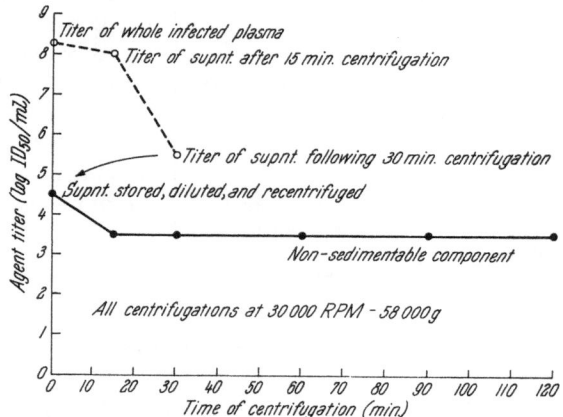

Fig. 21. Diagram showing the LDV titre in the supernatant after centrifugation of an LDV preparation and recentrifugation of the supernatant. (From RILEY, 1968b)

diameter of 35 to 40 nm. These data are not in themselves very convincing, since the recorded reduction in titre following centrifugation shows that 99.99 per cent of the viral infectivity is sedimentable, and as NOTKINS (1965a) has pointed out, the residual 'non-sedimentable' infectivity may represent part of a normal distribution curve, or a procedural artifact. But two other pieces of evidence have been produced in support of the two particle hypothesis. ADAMS and BOWMAN (1964) found that the proportion of viral infectivity that was non-sedimentable was higher at 14 days than at 1 day after infection, and also reported that viral infectivity from plasma taken at these two time points eluted differently from columns of DEAE-cellulose. CRISPENS (1964c) reported that the sedimentable, but not the non-sedimentable virus, was inactivated by heating to 50° C in 1 M $MgCl_2$, and using this difference as an assay for small and large particles he also reached the conclusion that the proportion of non-sedimentable particles increased during infection (STARK and CRISPENS, 1965). By 7 weeks, all the viral infectivity resisted heating to 50° C in $MgCl_2$, and was assumed to be due to small particles (Fig. 22).

Although these results strongly suggest that there are two groups of infectious LDV particles which differ in certain physical properties, the conclusion that they represent small and large particles is probably incorrect. Not only has it not been possible to demonstrate the presence of particles smaller than 45 nm by careful Gradocol filtration studies (ROWSON, MAHY, and SALAMAN, 1963; NOTKINS and SHOCHAT, 1963; DU BUY and JOHNSON, 1965), but neither has any difference in size been demonstrable by filtration between virus prepared at 1 and at 72 days after infection (Rowson, unpublished observations—Table 4). The radiation target size of the nucleic acid core of LDV has also been determined: there was no evidence of any variation in size of the nucleic acid core, and the kinetics of inactivation of 1 and 72 day virus were the same (Fig. 23) (Rowson, Parr, and Alper, 1968a and b). A more likely explanation for the alteration in properties of LDV during the course of infection is a change in the surface properties of the particle

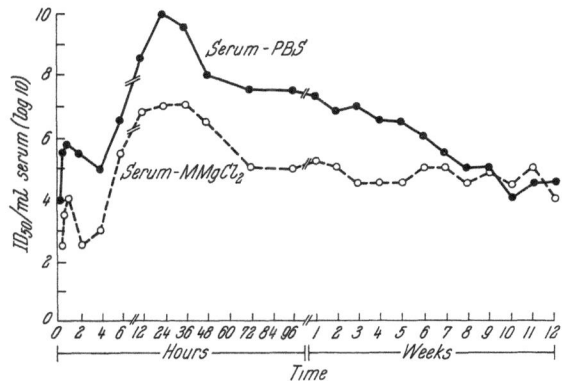

Fig. 22. Plasma LDV titre in mice following the injection of LDV.
Titre measured directly and after heating in the presence of 2 M magnesium chloride. The proportion of heat labile virus falls after prolonged infection. (From Stark and Crispens, 1965)

brought about by the presence of a blocking antibody on the surface of the virus from chronically infected mice (Notkins, Mahar, Scheele, and Goffman, 1966), or the enclosure of the virion within a single or double membraned lipid-containing vesicle (Du Buy and Johnson, 1965). A surface change brought about by either method would provide an explanation for the increase in resistance to neutralization by LDV antiserum shown by virus occurring in plasma late in infection (see p. 78).

Table 4. *Infectivity before and after Filtration of LDV Prepared from Mice Infected for 1 or 100 Days*

| Average pore diameter of Gradocol membrane | 1 day virus Virus titre ($\log_{10}$) | | 100 day virus Virus titre ($\log_{10}$) | |
|---|---|---|---|---|
| | before | after | before | after |
| 87 nm | 4.0 | $<1$ | 3.0 | $<1$ |
| 220 nm | 2.5 | 2.5 | 5.0 | 4.0 |

In summary, whilst there is some evidence that LDV particles of differing surface properties occur in mouse plasma during infection, there is no conclusive evidence for the existence of infectious particles of widely differing size.

Studies on the behaviour of infectious LDV on density gradients have been carried out by four groups of workers. Mahy (1963) subjected mouse plasma preparations containing LDV to centrifugation in a 2 M caesium chloride solution at 36,000 r.p.m. (130,000 $g$) for 24 hours in the SW 39 L Spinco rotor. Virus infectivity was recovered in a broad band at densities of 1.168 to 1.180 under these conditions. RILEY (1968b) reported experiments in which LDV was centrifuged on a 0 to 70 per cent sucrose gradient at 136,000 × $g$ for 1, 16, 40 and 85 hours. It was concluded from these experiments that the bulk of the virus sedimented at a density of 1.168. NOTKINS and his colleagues (NOTKINS, 1971a; NIWA, YAMAZAKI, BADER, and NOTKINS, 1973) grew radioactively-labelled LDV in mouse embryo cultures treated with $^3$H uridine, and centrifuged the 300-fold concentrated culture supernatants on a 10—60 per cent linear sucrose gradient for 20 hours at 100,000 × $g$. He also obtained a peak of infectivity at 1.17 g/ml and this coincided with the peak radioactivity. Cultures labelled with $^3$H thymidine did not give such a radioactive peak in the infectivity band.

DARNELL and PLAGEMANN (1972) isolated LDV labelled with $^3$H uridine from mouse peritoneal macrophage culture fluid by isopycnic centrifugation in linear sucrose density gradients (0.5 to 1.5 M sucrose). The density of the virus was estimated to be 1.12 g/ml from the coincidence of infectivity and radioactivity at this position in the gradient after centrifugation for 14 hours. The experiment was controlled by similar studies on the L-cell-associated oncornavirus which had a density of 1.16 g/ml; Newcastle disease virus (1.19 g/ml); vesicular stomatitis virus (1.19 g/ml) and Sindbis virus (1.18 g/ml). The reason for the lower density of LDV in these experiments compared to previous reports was attributed by DARNELL and PLAGEMANN (1972) to a relatively greater lipid content in their virus, perhaps the result of a more gentle isolation procedure than that used by other workers, since in some circumstances (with 0.5 per cent pancreatic autolysate in the culture medium) infectious LDV of density 1.16 g/ml was recovered. However, when they examined a preparation of LDV obtained from Notkins' laboratory, this virus also sedimented at a density of 1.12 g/ml (DARNELL, personal communication). Further studies of the physical properties of LDV seem warranted.

The nucleic acid component of LDV is ribonucleic acid (RNA). This was first demonstrated by NOTKINS and SCHEELE (1963a) who used plasma from mice infected for 24 hours which had an infectious titre of $10^{10.5}$ ID$_{50}$/ml on titration using intracerebral or intramuscular injection into test mice. The extract was inactivated in 20 minutes at room temperature by pancreatic ribonuclease (10 µg/ ml) but not by deoxyribonuclease (300 µg/ml). Subsequently, it was reported that infectious ribonucleic acid could also be obtained from LDV by extraction with butanol, chloroform, or ether (NOTKINS, 1964a and b, 1965c). The results with ether were particularly surprising since it had already been reported that the infectivity of intact LDV was lost following treatment with ether (NOTKINS and SHOCHAT, 1963). This suggested that the effect of ether treatment of the whole virus might be to alter the structure of the viral envelope in such a way as to prevent entry into the host cell, in this case it should still be possible to extract an infectious nucleic acid from ether-inactivated virus by the GIERER and SCHRAMM (1956) method. However, all attempts in this direction were unsuccessful (NOTKINS, 1964a) and as an alternative explanation for the ether sensitivity it was postulated that damage to the viral envelope by ether might expose the viral nucleic acid to nucleases present in the medium. NOTKINS (1964a) showed that LDV was inactivated by ether in the presence of plasma, but that, if the virus was first separated from plasma and suspended in ribonuclease-free medium, infectivity was partly resistant to ether treatment. The presence of tissue nucleases may also explain the earlier failure of the Munich group to extract an infectious nucleic acid from LDV-infected mouse tissues (BRDICZKA, GEORGII, and ZOBL, 1963). Another factor to be considered is the presence of heparin which NOTKINS and COSMIDES (1964) have shown to inactivate the viral nucleic acid.

The preparation of infectious ribonucleic acid from LDV is interesting since it has generally proved difficult, if not impossible, to obtain an infectious nucleic acid from other ether-sensitive RNA viruses such as the influenza, parainfluenza,

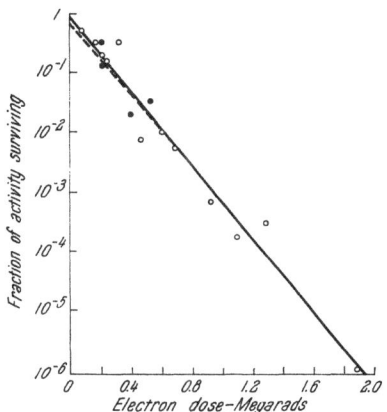

Fig. 23. Kinetics of inactivation of LDV.
Survival of virus from mice 24 hours (O) and 72 days (●) after infection. Points from 3 experiments using 24 hour virus and 2 experiments using 72 day virus. The solid and broken lines have been drawn to give the best fit (method of least squares) to the data for the 24 hour and 72 day virus, respectively. There is no significant difference in the survival curve parameters. (From ROWSON, PARR, and ALPER, 1968)

rhabdovirus and RNA tumour virus groups (SCHAFFER, 1962). Only from the ether-sensitive arboviruses, both groups A and B, can infectious RNA be readily obtained (CHENG, 1958; ANDERSON and ADA, 1959), and as with LDV, it has been found that removal of the outer coat, e.g. with deoxycholate, releases infectious ribonucleic acid provided care is taken to avoid exposure to serum or tissue ribonucleases (RICHTER and WECKER, 1963).

The ability of free viral RNA to infect cells implies that the nucleic acid of LDV can function directly as a messenger RNA without the need for prior synthesis of a complementary strand (BALTIMORE, 1971). Thus, the virion would not be expected to contain an RNA-dependent RNA transcriptase; the absence of detectable virion transcriptase activity in LDV has been reported by DARNELL and PLAGEMANN (1972). Tests for reverse transcriptase (RNA-dependent DNA polymerase) activity were also reported to be negative (NOTKINS, 1971a).

If LDV does indeed bear a close relationship with viruses of the togavirus group, as its overall size and the infectivity of the viral RNA would imply, there should be a similarity to other togaviruses in the size and amount of RNA in the virus particle. Semliki Forest virus, a group A togavirus, contains $4.1 \times 10^6$ daltons of RNA, which constitutes some 5 per cent of the particle weight (KENNEDY and BURKE, 1972).

Information on the size of LDV-RNA has been obtained indirectly by measurement of the radiation target size. Rowson, Parr, and Alper (1968a and b) exposed freeze-dried preparations of LDV in air to the electron beam from a linear accelerator to find the radiation target size of the nucleic acid core (see Fig. 23). The straight line fitted to the exponential points yields a value of 0.14 megarads for the value of the dose which gives survival $e^{-1}$, i.e. the dose needed to give an average of one lethal event per particle with 95 per cent confidence limits of 0.12 to 0.16 megarads. According to the calculations of Lea (1946), the corresponding confidence limits for the molecular weight of the nucleic acid core are 6 to $8 \times 10^6$ daltons. Ginoza (1967) compared the estimates of the size of nucleic acid cores obtained by irradiation and other methods and concluded that the agreement was good for RNA and single stranded DNA viruses, but that for double stranded DNA viruses the radiation target size was in general too small. On the basis of Ginoza's review, the value of 6 to $8 \times 10^6$ daltons for LDV nucleic acid is unlikely to be too high. However, the relationship between the molecular weight and the size of the whole virus measured by filtration suggests that it may indeed be an overestimate. A single-stranded RNA molecule of this size could code for some twenty average-sized polypeptides, whereas the group A togaviruses, of similar overall size to LDV, contain only two structural proteins, one associated with the core and the other with the viral envelope while the group B togaviruses contain one core and two envelope proteins.

The possibility that LDV contains a partially double-stranded RNA genome is worth considering though this is unlikely since infectious LDV-RNA is sensitive to ribonuclease (Notkins, 1964a). A number of viruses of the arbovirus type have been identified which can be distinguished from the togaviruses on the basis of various physical criteria, but which form a distinct group having double-stranded RNA genomes (Borden, Shope, and Murphy, 1971). Included in this group are bluetongue, rabbit syncytium, equine encephalosis, Colorado tick fever, and African louse sickness viruses.

The most direct indication of the possible double-stranded nature of LDV nucleic acid would be analysis for base composition (Green, 1965). Approximate pairing between the amounts of guanine and cytosine, and adenosine and uracil, would suggest a double-stranded structure. However, the only relevant report is that of Adams and Bowman (1964) who compared the base composition of a high speed centrifuge pellet from infected mouse plasma, infective titre $10^{11}$ $ID_{50}$/ml, with the base composition of a similar pellet from normal mouse plasma. The amount of RNA present was found to be 40 µg/100 ml in normal plasma and 60 µg/100 ml in LDV-infected plasma. The base composition of normal plasma RNA was adenine, 23.0 per cent, guanine, 34.5 per cent, cytidine, 23.0 per cent, and uridine, 19.5 per cent; the base composition of the RNA derived from infected plasma did not differ significantly from these values (Adams and Bowman, 1964). However, no conclusions can be drawn from this experiment; it will be necessary to extract RNA from virus which has been adequately purified and is known to be free of cellular material before the base composition of LDV-RNA can be determined.

Recently, Darnell and Plagemann (1972 and 1973) have estimated the sedimentation coefficient of LDV-RNA from virions grown in mouse macrophage cultures in the presence of $^3$H-uridine as 48 S, relative to Sindbis virus as 43 S.

This would give the LDV genome a molecular weight of $5 \times 10^6$ daltons, from the formula of SPIRIN (1963). The RNA was not sensitive to heat treatment under conditions which revealed the subunit structure of L cell oncornavirus-RNA, and was completely sensitive to ribonuclease. DARNELL and PLAGEMANN (1972) concluded that LDV contains a single-stranded RNA molecule composed of a continuous polynucleotide chain. NIWA, YAMAZAKI, BADER, and NOTKINS (1973) estimated the molecular weight of LDV-RNA by its mobility after electrophoresis in agarose-polyacrylamide composite gels. The RNA extracted from the virus banded in a sucrose density gradient at 1.16 to 1.18 g per ml. A single peak migrated more slowly than the 45 S RNA marker. By extrapolation from the known molecular weight of the marker they estimated the molecular weight of LDV-RNA to be $6 \times 10^6$ daltons. This is in good agreement with the radiation inactivation data.

There are reports from at least one laboratory (NOTKINS, 1971a; YAMAZAKI and NOTKINS, 1973) that the replication of LDV is sensitive to pre-treatment of the cells with actinomycin D, an inhibitor of DNA-dependent RNA synthesis. This would imply, since the virus was not similarly sensitive to inhibitors of DNA synthesis such as cytosine-β-D arabinofuranoside and 5-fluorodeoxyuridine (NOTKINS, 1971a; YAMAZAKI and NOTKINS, 1973), that LDV requires host DNA-dependent RNA synthesis during the early stages of replication. At least one togavirus, Japanese B encephalitis, has been shown to be sensitive to actinomycin D (ZEBOVITZ, LEONG, and DOUGHTY, 1972). HOWEVER, both DU BUY and JOHNSON (1970) and EVANS (1970) found no significant effect of actinomycin D on LDV replication, and until the recent reports of NOTKINS (1971a) and YAMAZAKI and NOTKINS (1973) are confirmed, further speculation on this point would seem unwarranted.

Recently, the polypeptides of LDV grown in primary mouse peritoneal macrophage cultures have been analyzed by polyacrylamide gel electrophoresis (MICHAELIDES and SCHLESINGER, 1973). Three proteins were identified in the virion with estimated molecular weight of 13,000, 17,000 and 28,000, respectively. The 13,000 molecular weight protein was associated with the viral nucleocapsid and the other two proteins with the envelope. Similar sized polypeptides have been reported to occur in group B togaviruses (WESTAWAY, 1973). These results, coupled with the evidence on the size and morphology of the infectious particle, its sensitivity to lipid solvents, and the ability of extracted RNA to initiate infection, all suggest that LDV should be classified as a togavirus. However, the size of the viral RNA, whether estimated by radiation target size (ROWSON, PARR, and ALPER, 1968), zonal sedimentation (DARNELL and PLAGEMANN, 1972), or gel electrophoresis (NIWA, YAMAZAKI, BADER, and NOTKINS, 1973) appears to be considerably higher than that of known togaviruses; further studies will be necessary before LDV can be assigned to this or any other virus group.

## C. Antigenic Structure

The final identification of a virus usually depends on its antigenic structure, and in some cases several serological types of a particular virus can be recognized. The study of the antigenic structure of LDV has proved difficult because conventional neutralization tests in which the virus is mixed with antiserum and the mixture tested for infectivity fail to show inactivation of the virus (DU BUY and JOHNSON, 1965). This, combined with the permanent viraemia seen in LDV infected mice, suggested that antibodies were not being formed and led to doubts about the antigenicity of the virus. However, it proved possible to demonstrate the presence of neutralizing antibodies in the plasma of infected mice if a fall in virus titre was looked for rather than complete neutralization and if the test virus was obtained from mice infected for only a few days (ROWSON, MAHY, and BENDINELLI, 1966; NOTKINS, MAHAR, SCHEELE, and GOFFMAN, 1966). That virus in the plasma of chronically infected mice is resistant to neutralization with LDV antiserum is an interesting phenomenon further discussed on p. 78. It appears to result from the formation of virus-antibody complexes which are infectious but resistant to neutralization by further exposure to anti-viral serum.

Although LDV antibodies can be demonstrated by the indirect fluorescent antibody technique 6 days after infection, their titre rises slowly not reaching a maximum before 28 days (PORTER, PORTER, and DEERHAKE, 1969). Neutralizing activity is also slow to develop and could not be demonstrated in mouse plasma until 34 days post-infection (ROWSON, MAHY, and BENDINELLI, 1966). The plasma of LDV-infected mice always contains infective virus which must be inactivated or removed by filtration before the serum can be used in neutralization tests. This complication could be avoided by preparing antisera in another species. BAILEY and his colleagues (BAILEY, CLOUGH, LOHAUS, and WRIGHT, 1965) used rats and immunized them by the intraperitoneal injection of virus but they give no details of their immunization procedure or the kinetics of the antibody response. That antibodies to LDV are produced in rats and hamsters following an injection of virus receives support from experiments in which viral infectivity disappeared from the plasma slightly faster after a second injection of LDV than after a primary injection. The effect was most marked during the early part of the experiment as there appeared to be a residue of virus which was resistant to removal, and infectivity persisted for the same length of time following the first and second injections of virus (RILEY, 1968b).

All the strains of LDV so far tested behave in the same way on injection into mice and produce identical changes in plasma enzyme levels (POPE and ROWE, 1964; BAILEY and WRIGHT, 1965). Their antigenic properties have received little attention but BAILEY and his colleagues (BAILEY, CLOUGH, LOHAUS, and WRIGHT, 1965) found that one strain was more susceptible to neutralization by a rat antiserum prepared against the homologous virus than by antisera prepared against seven other strains. This work has not been extended or repeated by others and in view of the difficulties in comparing partial neutralization tests it should not be taken as proved that LDV strains differ antigenically. One source of error in comparing virus preparations is that the proportion of unneutralizable virus increases with time after infection (ROWSON, MAHY, and BENDINELLI, 1966). Over 90 per cent of the infectivity in virus preparations obtained from mice during the first few days of infection will be neutralized on exposure to antiserum but in chronically infected mice the virus will be completely resistant. It is therefore advisable to use virus from mice infected for only 24 hours in any neutralization tests in which different virus strains are being compared.

Of the other serological tests that have been used in the study of the antigenic structure of viruses none have been applied to LDV except for one report that antiserum prepared against bee chronic paralysis virus did not react with LDV in an Ouchterlony gel diffusion test (GIBBS, 1969).

## D. Resistance to Physical and Chemical Agents

The rather laborious nature of the methods for titrating LDV have made workers reluctant to devote their limited resources to compiling detailed studies of inactivation of LDV by physical and chemical agents. However, there are several observations recorded in the literature and from these LDV would appear to be an ether-sensitive virus with no unusual resistance or susceptibility to physical or chemical agents.

### 1. Temperature

Stock preparations of LDV consisting of pooled mouse plasma may be stored at —70° C or lower indefinitely, with virtually no loss of infectivity; freezing and thawing has little deleterious effect (NOTKINS and SHOCHAT, 1963). RILEY (1968b) has studied the survival of LDV at 4° and —20° C. At 4° C there was a slow loss of infectivity, the titre falling by 3.5 logs in 32 days. At —20° C there was a 2 log loss of infectivity in one month but no further loss was observed in the subsequent 5 months. LDV is sufficiently stable at room temperature for it to be manipulated without significant inactivation during short-term experimental operations of up to 24 hours (NOTKINS, 1965a). Infected faeces at room temperature lose infectivity between 96 and 120 hours (CRISPENS, 1964b). At higher temperatures the virus loses infectivity rapidly. There is a number of reports describing a loss of titre of two logs or more after incubation of the virus at 37° C for 24 hours, and complete inactivation within 48 hours at this temperature (BAYERLE, GEORGII, and JAKOB, 1962; NOTKINS and SHOCHAT, 1963; EVANS and SALAMAN, 1965; RILEY, 1968b). This raises problems in interpreting the infective titres of LDV released into the medium of tissue cultures maintained at 37° C. Detailed studies on the rates of inactivation of LDV diluted in tissue culture medium have shown that virus titres of $10^{4.5}$ $ID_{50}$ per ml or less are inactivated within 24 hours at 37° C (EVANS and SALAMAN, 1965).

The inactivation temperature of LDV infectivity during brief periods of heating (up to 30 minutes) is close to 60° C (CRISPENS, 1965a; RILEY, 1963b; BAILEY, STEARMAN, and CLOUGH, 1963; NOTKINS and SHOCHAT, 1963) and the virus can be completely inactivated by heating at 58° C for one hour (BAILEY, STEARMAN, and CLOUGH, 1963; ROWSON, MAHY, and BENDINELLI, 1966) which does not destroy the neutralizing antibodies present in infected mouse plasma. Boiling for 2 minutes destroys the infectivity of LDV (NOTKINS and SHOCHAT, 1963).

In the presence of magnesium chloride, LDV is more sensitive to heat inactivation at 50° C (CRISPENS, 1965a). Stability of certain enteroviruses to heat (50° C) in the presence of 1 M $MgCl_2$ was first demonstrated by WALLIS and MELNICK (1962), and it was found that some picornaviruses, such as rhinoviruses are inactivated under these conditions (DIMMOCK and TYRRELL, 1964) whereas others, such as echoviruses, are not (WALLIS and MELNICK, 1962). In the case of LDV, STARK and CRISPENS (1965) showed that sensitivity to heat inactivation in 1 M MgCl$_2$ depended on the time following infection at which the virus was harvested. Virus harvested at 24—48 hours post-infection was more resistant to heat inactivation (50° C for 60 minutes in 1 M MgCl$_2$) than virus harvested at 10—14 days or later. The evidence as to whether this results from the existence of two types of LDV particles has been discussed earlier (p. 32).

## 2. pH and Dilution Medium

LDV withstands variations in pH of the suspending medium from pH 6 to pH 8 with no loss of infectivity (RILEY, 1968 b). Considerable inactivation occurs if the virus is suspended in acid (pH 3) media (CRISPENS, 1965a), whereas it is relatively stable at pH 10.3 (NOTKINS and SHOCHAT, 1963).

NOTKINS and SHOCHAT (1963) compared a number of diluents (Eagle's MEM supplemented with 20 per cent veal infusion broth, phosphate buffered saline, distilled water, citrate-phosphate and carbonate buffers), exposing the virus diluted 1:100 to the diluent for 3 hours at 4° C before titration. They obtained the highest virus titres using Eagle's MEM with 20 per cent veal infusion broth.

RILEY (1968 b) reports a detailed study of the effects of various dilution media on LDV, and found that it was possible to use ordinary 0.9 per cent sodium chloride as a diluent provided the preparation was injected within one hour. Addition of 5 per cent calf serum to the saline medium greatly improves the stability of the virus, but there is a danger that repeated injections of heterologous serum at this concentration may cause anaphylactic shock. For this reason, a lower concentration of serum, 0.5 to 1 per cent, is recommended as a protectant (RILEY, 1968 b).

## 3. Chemicals

Intact LDV is inactivated on exposure to lipid solvents such as ether, chloroform or butanol. The classical test for ether sensitivity is exposure to 20 per cent diethyl ether at 4° C overnight (ANDREWES and HORSTMANN, 1949); these conditions completely inactivate LDV (NOTKINS and SHOCHAT, 1963; CRISPENS, 1965; MAHY, HARVEY, and ROWSON, 1966). Chloroform has greater polarity as a lipid solvent than ether and is probably a better substance to use for testing for the presence of essential lipid in viruses (FELDMAN and WANG, 1961). Treatment with chloroform (5 per cent) for 10 minutes at room temperature completely inactivates LDV (MAHY, HARVEY, and ROWSON, 1966), as does shaking with an equal volume of chloroform or butanol for 7 minutes at room temperature (NOTKINS and SHOCHAT, 1963). Less polar solvents, such as petroleum ether, may be used to extract from the virus some lipids which are apparently non-essential for infectivity. Figure 24 shows an electron micrograph of virus partially purified using petroleum ether (DU BUY and JOHNSON, 1965). NOTKINS (1965 c) has presented evidence that lipid solvents are only completely effective in causing inactivation of LDV provided ribonuclease is present in the virus suspension. If care is taken to avoid the presence of contaminating ribonuclease (present in normal mouse plasma), the chloroform or butanol treatment results in release of infectious RNA from the virion.

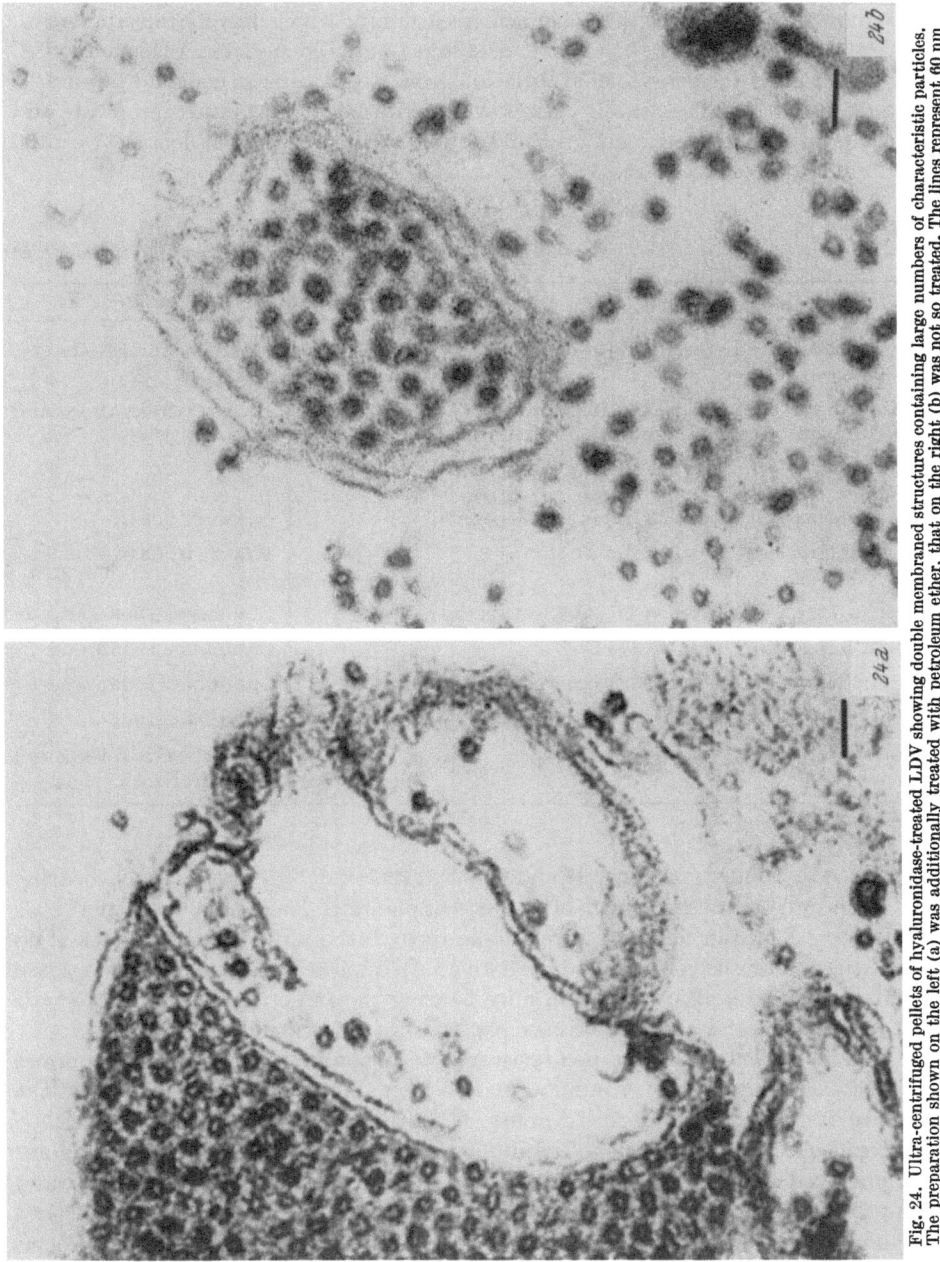

Fig. 24. Ultra-centrifuged pellets of hyaluronidase-treated LDV showing double membraned structures containing large numbers of characteristic particles. The preparation shown on the left (a) was additionally treated with petroleum ether, that on the right (b) was not so treated. The lines represent 60 nm

## 4. Miscellaneous Physical and Chemical Treatments

A number of physical and chemical treatments which have been applied to LDV are listed in Table 5. CRISPENS (1965a) exposed infected plasma at 8° C in a watch glass to ultraviolet irradiation from a Sylvania germicidal lamp at a distance of 14 cm. The watch glasses were agitated at 10 minute intervals and the virus titrated at intervals up to 90 minutes. Infectivity was lost between 60 and 90 minutes of exposure.

Table 5. *Inactivation of LDV by Various Physical and Chemical Procedures (See also Text)*

| Procedure | Inactivation | Reference |
|---|---|---|
| Lyophilization and storage at 4° or 22° C for 90 days | — | NOTKINS and SHOCHAT, 1963 |
| Antibiotic mixture (penicillin 100 units, streptomycin 50 mg/ml, acromycin 50 mg/ml and mycostatin 50 mg/ml) injected (IP) daily for 5 days | — | BAILEY, STEARMAN and CLOUGH, 1963 |
| Ribonuclease 100 μg/ml, 23 hours at 23°—25° C | — | RILEY, 1968b |
| Deoxyribonuclease 100 μg/ml, 23 hours at 23° to 25° C | — | RILEY, 1968b |
| Trypsin 5 mg/ml, 1 hour at 37° C | — | CRISPENS, 1965a and c |
| Papain 5 mg/ml, 1 hour at 37° C | — | CRISPENS, 1965a and c |
| Sodium deoxycholate 1:1000, 1 hour at 37° C | ± | CRISPENS, 1965a and c |
| Formalin 1:2500, 12 hours at 4° C | ± | CRISPENS, 1965a and c |
| Alcohol | + | GEORGII, GOLDBRUNNER and BRDICZKA, 1964 |

NOTKINS, BERRY, MOLONEY, and GREENFIELD (1962) exposed mice bearing the LDV-infected ascitic form of P-388 lymphocytic leukaemia to 10,000 rads whole body X-irradiation and were able to recover the virus from the ascitic fluid free of the tumour cells which had been killed. In another experiment they exposed freshly aspirated ascitic fluid from mice bearing the same tumour to $5 \times 10^6$ rads of X-irradiation and after this treatment no infectivity could be recovered.

CRISPENS (1965a) also studied resistance to formalin, by mixing four volumes of infected plasma with 1 volume of 1:500 formalin solution and incubated the mixture at 4° C and pH 7.2 for 72 hours. The titre fell slowly from 7.5 to 5.0 $ID_{50}$/ml. He also exposed the virus to sodium deoxycholate 1:1000 at 37°C for one hour and observed a fall in titre from 6.5 to 3.5 $ID_{50}$/ml. GEORGII, GOLDBRUNNER, and BRDICZKA (1964), found LDV to be inactivated by p-aminosalicyclic acid, and under certain conditions not stated, RILEY (1968b) reports that the virus is sensitive to chloromycetin (chloramphenicol). He found that chloromycetin administered daily to mice caused a fall in virus titre and their LDH activity failed to increase in the usual manner following infection. As might be expected, aureomycin and terramycin have no effect (RILEY, 1968b).

EBERT, CHIRIGOS, and ELLSWORTH (1968) studied the effects of chemotherapy with streptonigrin (4 daily subcutaneous injections of 0.3 mg/kg) or 6-mercapto-purine (4 daily subcutaneous injections of 60 mg/kg) from 4 to 7 days after LDV infection. No effects on plasma LDH levels of the mice were observed up to 20 days post-infection, and the drugs did not reduce plasma virus titres below control levels on days 8 or 14.

# V. Cultivation of the Virus

## A. Mice

The LDV replicates with remarkable speed in mice. The growth curve (Fig. 4) shows the rapid rise in titre of infective virus in the plasma during the first 24 hours after infection. A peak level is reached after 24 hours even when a small dose of virus is injected. Figure 25 shows the virus titre in the plasma during the first

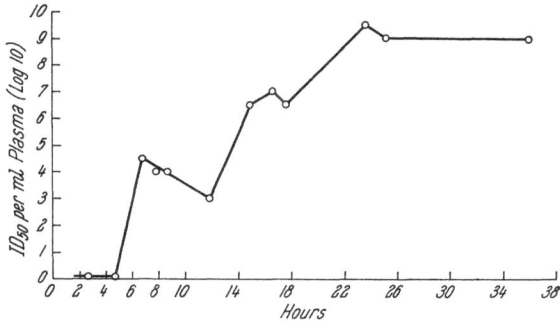

Fig. 25. Titre of LDV in the plasma of mice following the intraperitoneal injection of 100 ID₅₀ of LDV

36 hours after the injection of 100 ID$_{50}$ of LDV. There is a latent period of five hours followed by a sudden rise in plasma virus titre. There is then no further increase in virus titre until the end of a second latent period which lasts five to six hours. The stepwise growth curve suggests that virus must be released very rapidly from the infected cells perhaps with their destruction, but no morphological lesions have been observed in histological studies to confirm this.

## 1. Site of Replication

In an attempt to determine where virus replication was taking place, we infected mice with a small number (five to ten) of infective doses of virus and tested various organs such as liver, spleen and kidney for virus five hours after the injection, but were unable to demonstrate the presence of any in the tissues before it appeared in the plasma (ROWSON, 1964). DU BUY and JOHNSON (1966) assayed various tissues for virus infectivity twenty-four hours after LDV infection (Table 6) and found that the spleen, superficial lymph nodes and thymus had titres approaching that in the plasma, whereas the liver, kidneys, pancreas and brain had lower titres. Perfusion of the spleen and lymph nodes before titration did

not reduce the virus titre and they considered that the virus in these tissues was
not wholly due to the presence of plasma. In the tissues where they had found the
greatest amount of virus (spleen, lymph nodes and thymus) they followed the rise
in virus titre during the first 48 hours after infection. The rise in titre in these tissues
coincided with that in the plasma, and the titre in the lymph nodes 18, 24 and
36 hours after infection was higher than in the plasma. In electron microscopic

Table 6. *Concentration of LDV in Various Tissues 16 or 24 Hours after Infection*

| Tissue | Virus titre ($\log_{10}$ $ID_{50}$/ml) | |
|--------|-----------------------------------------|---|
|        | PLAGEMANN, GREGORY, SWIM and CHAN (1963) | DU BUY and JOHNSON (1966) |
| Plasma | 8.3 | 10.0 |
| Spleen | 8.0 | 10.5 |
| Lymph nodes | — | 9.9 |
| Thymus | — | 9.8 |
| Liver | 8.0 | 9.0 |
| Kidney | 7.0 | 8.5 |
| Pancreas | — | 8.5 |
| Brain | 6.7 | 7.5 |
| Small intestine | 7.7 | — |
| Urinary bladder | 6.0 | — |

studies of lymph nodes and spleens up to 24 hours after infection, they were only
able to find virus particles in large numbers in the cytoplasm of certain lymph node
cells. BAILEY and MONROE (1972) have reported that the virus titre in lymph nodes
is higher than in the plasma 24 to 48 hours after infection. PLAGEMANN and his
colleagues (PLAGEMANN, GREGORY, SWIM, and CHAN, 1963) also titrated the virus
content of various tissues (Table 6) and found sixteen hours after infection that
the spleen and liver had the same virus titre as the plasma whereas the lungs,
kidneys, small intestine and brain had lower titres. They did not examine the
thymus and lymph nodes. In order to determine the nature of the cells in which the
virus was replicating, DU BUY and JOHNSON (1966) irradiated mice with 900 r
whole body X-irradiation and infected them 48 hours later. The lymphocyte count
in the blood was reduced by 99 per cent but the number of macrophages in the
peritoneal fluid was not reduced significantly and the virus titre in the plasma
24 hours after infection was as high as in unirradiated control animals. SNODGRASS,
LOWREY, and HANNA (1972) by electron microscopy were unable to find any
evidence of virus replication in the thymus except when the virus had been injected
directly into the thymus. They found virus particles in the marginal zone of
lymphoid nodules in the spleen and the medulla of the mesenteric lymph nodes
6 hours after infection. The number of virus particles had increased by 12 hours
and they were closely associated with the plasmalemma of reticular cells. At
this time, the virus particles were present in the thymus-dependent areas where
they were also associated with phagocytic reticular cells. Virus particles were not

seen in close relationship with lymphocytes, but there was evidence of an adverse effect on these cells. The cytotoxic effect on the lymphocytes was maximal at 2 days and subsided by 4 days after injection of LDV.

The LDV appears to replicate in radiation-resistant cells, probably macrophages, especially the phagocytic cells of the reticulum of the spleen and lymph nodes. This view receives some support from the studies on virus replication in tissue cultures (see p. 53) and from the fact that a large amount of virus is present in the ascitic

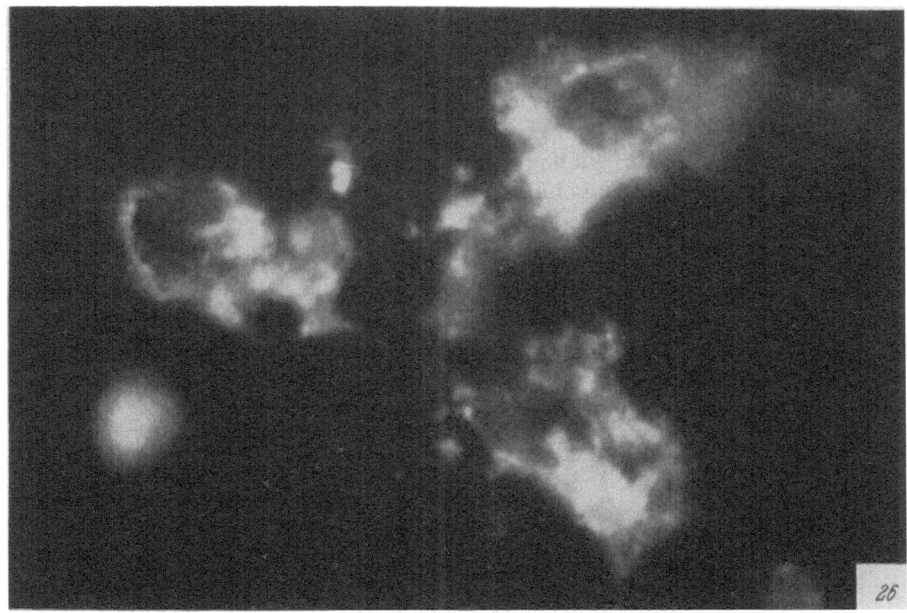

Fig. 26. Frozen section of spleen 24 hours after LDV injection.
Treated with mouse anti LDV serum and fluorochrome conjugated anti-mouse globulin

fluid of mice with the Ehrlich ascites carcinoma, 24 hours after infection with LDV (Du Buy and Johnson, 1965). The virus does not replicate in the tumour cells when these are grown in culture or in newborn rats, but if it is injected into the swollen peritoneal cavity of mice with ascites due to the tumour, the virus titre in the peritoneal cavity after 24 hours is comparable to that in the plasma. There is no reason to suppose that the virus is replicating in the tumour cells. It may be entering the peritoneal fluid from the plasma, but it seems likely that replication is taking place in the peritoneal macrophages.

Using the indirect fluorescent antibody technique, Porter, Porter, and Deerhake (1969) were able to demonstrate antigen-containing cells in sections of spleen and liver from mice infected 18 and 24 hours previously with LDV. Similar results were obtained by Rowson and Micheals (1973) (Fig. 26). No antigen-containing cells were seen in sections of kidney, lung, thymus or salivary gland. Porter and his colleagues did not examine sections of lymph nodes; there were more antigen-containing cells in the spleen than in the liver, so they examined spleen sections at intervals from 12 hours to 7 days after LDV infection. Twelve hours post-infection there was no definite staining. At 18 and 24 hours there were 1500 to 5000 stained cells per 6 to 8 square mm. By 36 hours, 200 or less cells were stained and there was a reduction in the number of nucleated cells in the red pulp of the spleen. Two days after infection and at times up to 7 days, antigen-containing cells were very few and difficult to identify. Such cells in the spleen were confined to the red pulp, and their appearance was compatible with their being macrophages. Antigen was mainly located in the cytoplasm and the slight nuclear staining observed may have been due to cytoplasm lying over or under the nucleus. In sections of liver 18 and 24 hours post-infection there were 100 to 400 antigen-containing cells per 25 square mm. There was no staining of liver cells, the staining being limited to Kupffer cells. Three days post-infection, the number of immunoglobulin-containing cells in the spleen was about twice the number seen in control mice, while at 4 and 7 days there were from 2 to 5 times the number. This increase in the immunoglobulin producing cells is in keeping with NOTKINS and his colleagues' observation of increased plasma gammaglobulin levels in LDV infected mice (NOTKINS, MERGENHAGEN, RIZZO, SCHEELE, and WALDMANN, 1966). It limited the usefulness of the indirect fluorescent antibody technique in the search for viral antigen in the later stages of infection, and using the direct method PORTER and his colleagues found the staining to be not very intense. These factors prevented the examination of chronically infected splenic tissue for viral antigen.

Table 7. *Effect of Nephrectomy on Replication of Lactic Dehydrogenase Virus*

| Treatment | Blood virus titre[a] ($\log_{10}$ $ID_{50}$/ml) Time after infection | |
|---|---|---|
| | 4 hours | 24 hours |
| None | 3.5 | 8.0 |
| Nephrectomized 2 hours after infection | | 3.0 |
| Nephrectomized 4 hours after infection | | 6.0 |

[a] All the mice were injected intravenously with the same dose of virus and the figures given are the means of 3 titrations using 2 mice at each 10-fold dilution.

ROWSON, MICHAELS and HURST (1974) made an electron microscopic study of the tissues of mice during the first few weeks after infection with LDV and found that there was a very early change in the kidney glomeruli (see p. 95). As early as 24 hours after infection there was swelling of the capillary endothelial cells, so there was a possibility that these changes might be due to virus replication in the capillary lining cells though no viral antigen could be demonstrated in these cells by immuno-fluorescence. To assess the role of the kidney cells in virus production, mice were bilaterally nephrectomized 2 or 4 hours after the injection of LDV intra-venously. As shown in Table 7, nephrectomy dramatically reduced the level of viraemia attained 24 hours after infection. Unfortunately, though mice appear quite normal for some hours after total nephrectomy, they are moribund after 22 hours and it is therefore difficult to be certain why nephrectomy reduces the virus titre at 24 hours after infection. That it is not due to removing the tissue in which the virus replicates is suggested by the fact that nephrectomy 4 hours after infection is very much less effective than nephrectomy 2 hours after infection. As no new virus is released before 5 hours after infection, one would expect removal of the tissue in which the virus replicates to be equally effective at 2 or 4 hours. The role of nephrectomy in reducing the level of viraemia requires further study.

## 2. Factors Affecting the Acute Phase of Infection

The rapid rise in virus titre during the first 24 hours after infection may be terminated by the action of interferon as high titres of interferon have been found in the plasma at this time (BARON, DU BUY, BUCKLER, and JOHNSON, 1964; BARON, BUCKLER, McCLOSKEY, and KIRSCHSTEIN, 1966; DU BUY and JOHNSON, 1965; FALKE and ROWE, 1965; EVANS and RILEY, 1968; DU BUY, BARON, UHLENDORF, and JOHNSON, 1973) and the virus is sensitive to the action of interferon (YAMAZAKI and NOTKINS, 1973; DU BUY, BARON, UHLENDORF, and JOHNSON, 1973). Support for the view that interferon production is responsible for controlling the very rapid virus replication taking place in the first day after infection comes from experiments using statolon, an interferon inducer and actinomycin D, which has been shown to inhibit the production of interferon in tissue cultures infected with the RNA of Chikungunya virus if added $1\frac{1}{2}$ hours or less after exposure to the virus (LEVY, AXELROD, and BARON, 1965). CRISPENS (1970a) found that the titre of LDV in the

Table 8. *The Effect of Various Substances on the Blood Virus Titre 24 Hours after the Injection of LDV*

| Test substance | Interval between injections of test substances and virus (hours) | Expected effect on RES | Level of viraemia 24 hours after virus injection ($\log_{10}$ ID$_{50}$ per ml blood) | |
|---|---|---|---|---|
| | | | Control | Test |
| Stilboestrol (implant) | 72 | Stimulation | 9.5[a] | 8.5 |
| (6 daily injections) | 48 | Stimulation | 8.5 | 8.5 |
| Carbon | 1 | Blockade | 10.0 | 10.5 |
| Zymosan | $\frac{1}{2}$ | Blockade | 9.0 | 10.0 |
| | 3 | Blockade | 9.0 | 10.0 |
| | 20 | Stimulation | 10.0 | 9.5 |
| Thorotrast | 1 | Blockade | 8.5 | 9.5 |
| | 18 | Blockade | 9.5 | 9.5 |

[a] Titrations performed using 2 mice at each 10-fold dilution. Values are the mean plasma virus titres of 2 mice.

plasma 24 hours after infection was significantly reduced by an intraperitoneal injection of 4.5 mg of statolon given between 6 and 12 hours before the virus. Given earlier or later it had less effect. He also found that the optimal dose was 4.5 mg and that it produced the most marked fall in titre when the infecting dose of virus was small. Actinomycin D, 10 mg injected intraperitoneally one hour before an injection of LDV, did not increase the plasma virus titre at 24 hours after infection, but higher virus titres were observed in the actinomycin D-treated mice than in control infected mice from 48 hours until one week after infection (CRISPENS, 1966a). If, in fact, interferon is responsible for terminating the rapid phase of virus production, some effect on the 24 hour virus titre should have been seen, but the drug may have been given too late. The mice were not examined to see if interferon production was in fact inhibited. An alternative explanation for the failure of interferon suppression by actinomycin D to increase the virus titre in the plasma may be that actinomycin D, as well as suppressing interferon production, also inhibits LDV replication (YAMAZAKI and NOTKINS, 1973).

Another factor which may be involved in terminating the rapid rise in virus titre is the death of available virus producing cells and a scarcity of further cells susceptible to infection.

It seems unlikely that the reticuloendothelial system plays any major role in limiting the peak level of viraemia as the administration of various substances which affect the phagocytic function of the reticuloendothelial system has no effect on the level of viraemia 24 hours after infection (ROWSON, MAHY, and SALAMAN, 1965). Table 8 shows the substances tested, their expected effect on the reticuloendothelial system and the 24 hour plasma virus titres in control and test mice.

### 3. Factors Affecting the Chronic Phase of Infection

Interferon may or may not play a part in terminating the phase of rapid virus production but it seems likely that it is at least partly responsible for the fairly rapid fall in plasma virus titre which occurs during the first week after infection (EVANS and RILEY, 1968). The plasma virus titre can be sharply reduced by the stimulation of interferon production (ROWSON, 1969). Figure 27 shows the plasma virus titre in three mice following the injection of statolon, an interferon stimulator. Within 48 hours of injection the level of viraemia fell by 2 to 3 $\log_{10}$ units but rapidly returned to the pre-treatment level. A similar observation has been made by CRISPENS (1970a). Du BUY and JOHNSON (1965) obtained a depression of plasma virus titre following the injection of $10^{8.5}$ PFU of Newcastle disease virus into mice 10 days after LDV infection.

Circulating antibodies appear late in the infection and presumably play no part in the fall in plasma virus titre during the first 2 to 3 weeks. However, it seems likely that they play a part in determining the stable level of viraemia after the first 3 weeks. Du BUY, WORTHINGTON, and JOHNSON (1971) followed the plasma virus titre in two groups of mice injected with LDV. One group was given weekly intraperitoneal injections of an immunosuppressive agent (cyclophosphamide, 75 mg per kg) commencing 12 hours after infection and continued for 24 weeks, while the other group received injections of phosphate buffered saline. For the first 2 to 3 weeks there was no significant difference between the plasma virus titre in the two groups but from the 4th week after infection until at least 28 weeks after cessation of drug treatment, the viraemia of the immuno-suppressed mice was about 1.0 to 2.5 $\log_{10}$ higher than in the control group.

In addition to neutralizing viral infectivity, antibodies may help in the removal of virus particles from the plasma by the reticuloendothelial system which consists of the fixed and wandering mononuclear phagocytic cells of the body (STUART, 1970). Although stimulation or blockade of the reticuloendothelial system had no effect on the peak level of viraemia 24 hours after infection, the stable level of virus in the plasma two weeks or more after infection is altered by the injection of substances which affect the phagocytic activity of the reticuloendothelial system (ROWSON, MAHY, and SALAMAN, 1965).

Figure 28 shows the rise in plasma virus titre which follows the intraperitoneal injection of a single dose of thorotrast, a potent reticuloendothelial blocking agent which reduces phagocytosis; and Figure 29 shows the small but prolonged depres-

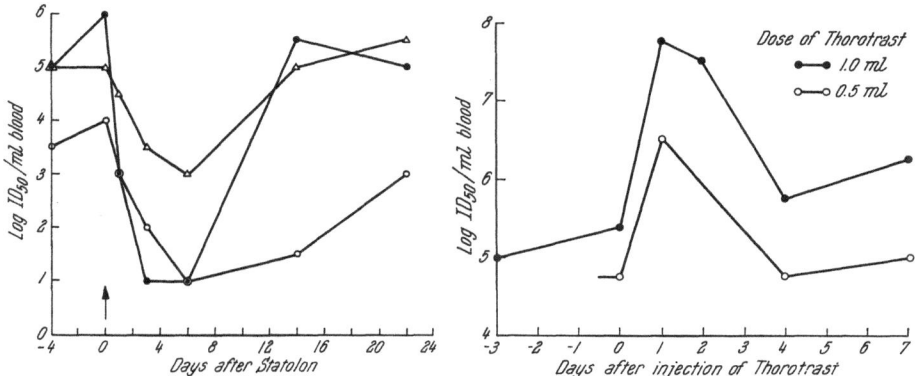

Fig. 27. Titre of LDV in the plasma of 3 mice following the injection of statolon

Fig. 28. Mean blood virus titre in 2 pairs of mice injected intraperitoneally with either 1.0 ml or 0.5 ml of thorotrast per mouse 10 days after infection with LDV. (From ROWSON, MAHY, and SALAMAN, 1965)

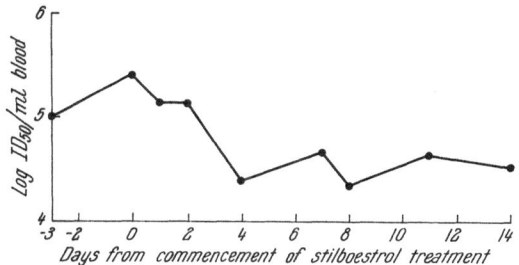

Fig. 29. Mean blood virus titre in 2 mice receiving a course of subcutaneous injections of stilboestrol. Six injections were given on days 0 to 5, each consisting of 0.1 mg stilboestrol/mouse, dissolved in 0.1 ml arachis oil. (From ROWSON, MAHY, and SALAMAN, 1965)

sion of the plasma virus titre following a course of subcutaneous injections of stilboestrol which stimulates the reticuloendothelial system. A single dose of zymosan at first blocks and then stimulates the reticuloendothelial system and Figure 30 shows the effect of zymosan on the level of viraemia. The rise in virus titre is not as great as that produced by thorotrast and the effect is shortlived. By 48 hours after injection the titre is depressed below the starting level. Rather surprisingly, bacterial endotoxin, a reticuloendothelial stimulating agent, did not significantly reduce the level of viraemia (ROWSON and MAHY, 1965).

Similar results have been reported in two other virus infections. Blockade of the reticuloendothelial system with thorotrast was found to increase the level of viraemia in mice infected with Semliki Forest virus (MIMS, 1964), and to decrease the rate at which injected Newcastle disease virus disappeared from the blood of mice (BRUNNER, HUREZ, McCLUSKEY, and BENACERRAF, 1960).

LDV-infected mice clear certain plasma enzymes more slowly than normal animals so it might be expected that they would be less efficient in clearing virus

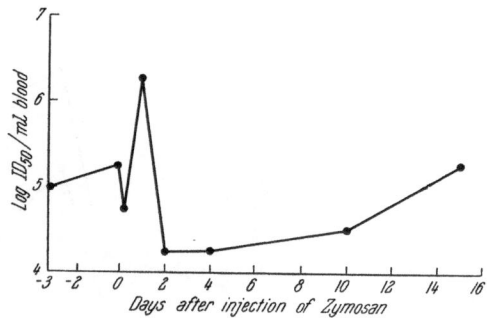

Fig. 30. Mean blood virus titre in 2 mice injected intravenously with zymosan (10 mg/100 g body weight as a suspension in normal saline) 10 days after infection with LDV. (From ROWSON, MAHY, and SALAMAN, 1965)

Table 9. *Clearance from the Plasma of Intravenously Injected LDV in Previously Uninfected Mice and in Mice Infected with LDV for 3 Weeks*

| Mouse No. | Previous LDV infection | Plasma virus titre[a] ($\log_{10}$ ID$_{50}$/ml) | |
| --- | --- | --- | --- |
| | | 2 minutes after virus injection | 3 hours after virus injection |
| 1 | — (no) | 8.5 | 7.3 |
| 2 | — (no) | 8.0 | 7.2 |
| 3 | — (no) | 8.5 | 7.0 |
| 4 | — (no) | 8.5 | 7.0 |
| Mean | | 8.4 | 7.2 |
| 5 | + (yes) | 7.7 | 6.5 |
| 6 | + (yes) | 8.3 | 6.3 |
| 7 | + (yes) | 7.8 | 7.0 |
| 8 | + (yes) | 8.5 | 5.9 |
| Mean | | 8.2 | 6.2 |

[a] Titrations performed using 6 mice at each 10-fold dilution.

particles also. It is not possible, strictly speaking, to measure the rate of LDV clearance from normal mice as the injected virus will initiate infection. However as no new virus is released into the plasma for 5 to 6 hours after infection, the clearance rate measured during this period in previously uninfected mice will be of injected virus only. We (ROWSON, MAHY, and SALAMAN, 1965) took two groups of four mice, one uninfected and the other infected with LDV twenty one days previously. All the mice were injected intravenously with 0.1 ml of a virus preparation containing $10^{9.5}$ $ID_{50}$ per ml. The mice were bled two minutes and three hours later and the virus titre in the plasma titrated. Table 9 shows the virus titres obtained. Since the dose of virus was large in comparison with the level of previously circulating virus in the infected mice it is not surprising that the virus titres in the two groups are virtually the same two minutes after injection. After three hours the mice previously infected had cleared rather more of the injected virus from their circulation than had the previously uninfected animals. It seems unlikely that antibody could have played any major role in the disappearance of viral infectivity as neutralizing antibodies are not demonstrable in the plasma as early as twenty-one days after infection. Further evidence that the reticuloendothelial system of mice chronically infected with LDV can clear particulate matter normally is the normal carbon clearance in such animals (MAHY, 1964) and the fact that bacteriophage $T_2$ is cleared normally (ROWSON and MAHY, 1965).

The stable and permanent viraemia in LDV infected mice does not appear to depend on blockade of the reticuloendothelial system and the available evidence suggests that there may be a quite rapid turnover of virus in the plasma. However, the clearance of antibody-stabilized virus has not been studied and it may be that this virus-antibody complex is not rapidly removed from the plasma.

### 4. Miscellaneous Substances Affecting the Growth of LDV

The action of a number of other substances on the replication of LDV have been reported.

Dimethyl benzanthracene has been reported to reduce interferon production *in vitro* (MAEYER and MAEYER-GUINGUARD, 1963). However, 0.4 mg suspended in 1 per cent gelatin and injected intraperitoneally into mice did not affect their response to LDV injected at time intervals from one hour to fourteen days later. Plasma virus titres twenty four hours after infection and LDH activity in the plasma at three days after infection were measured, but there was no difference between the control and dimethyl benzanthracene treated animals (ROWSON, 1963).

It has been suggested that 6-thioguanine is incorporated into the nucleic acid of cells and pretreatment with azaserine, an inhibiter of purine synthesis, enhances the inhibitory effect of 6-thioguanine. The action of these two substances on LDH virus replication was investigated by ADAMS and BOWMAN (1963). They took two groups of four mice and injected them with a small dose of LDV. Fifteen minutes previously one group had been given an intraperitoneal injection of 10 mg/kg of azaserine. One hour after infection this group was injected with 10 mg/kg of 6-thioguanine. The same dose was repeated at hourly intervals for 6 hours and finally two similar doses were given at 90 minute intervals. Blood was taken from the two groups 7, 11 and 24 hours after infection, and titrated in mice for infectivity. The treated group had lower plasma virus titres after 7 and 11 hours but by 24 hours both groups had titres of at least $10^7$ $ID_{50}$/ml. It seems possible that thioguanine may have been incorporated into the viral nucleic acid and delayed the production of infective virus during the period of administration, but the effect was shortlived.

The action of two other cancer chemotherapeutic agents, 6-mercaptopurine and streptonigrin has been investigated by EBERT, CHIRIGOS, and ELLSWORTH (1968). Both of these substances given daily for 4 days, commencing on the fourth day after Friend leukaemia virus infection, caused a 3 to 4 $\log_{10}$ reduction in the plasma virus titre until the 11th day after virus inoculation. After this, there was no significant difference between the treated and control mice. Similar treatment of LDV infected mice caused no alteration in plasma virus titre.

Orthophenarsine hydrochloride used to control *Eperythrozoon coccoides* infection has no effect on LDV replication (RILEY, LOVELESS, and FITZMAURICE, 1964).

## B. Other Animals

The LDV has not been shown to replicate in any species other than the mouse. PLAGEMANN and his colleagues (PLAGEMANN, GREGORY, SWIM, and CHAN, 1963) injected rats and golden Syrian hamsters with LDV but there was no elevation of the plasma LDH level and plasma taken from these animals one to two weeks after inoculation failed to infect mice on injection. NOTKINS (1965a) reports that the injection of LDV into rats, hamsters, guinea pigs and rabbits did not cause

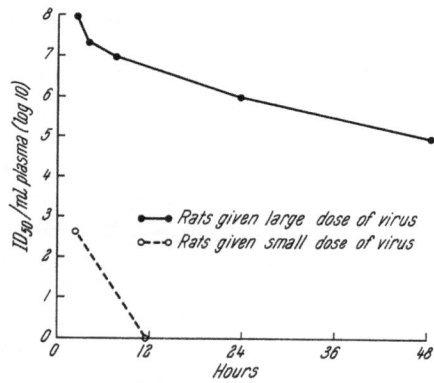

Fig. 31. Titre of LDV in the plasma of rats following intraperitoneal injection of infected mouse plasma

a rise in plasma LDH activity and attempts to demonstrate the virus in the plasma of these animals by injecting it into normal mice were unsuccessful. ROWSON (1966) injected deer mice *(peromyscus)* with LDV. After 5 minutes the plasma virus titre was $10^6$ $ID_{50}$/ml, but by 24 hours after injection no infective virus could be demonstrated. Figure 31 shows the steady fall in plasma virus titre in rats give a single injection of LDV. A small dose of virus has completely disappeared in 12 hours but with a larger dose some virus is still present in the plasma after 48 hours. Similar results were obtained by RAUEN and HUPE (1963). KAMPSCHMIDT, UPCHURCH, and JOHNSON (1966) could find no evidence for a LDV in rats, and this failure of LDV to replicate has been used as a method of freeing various tumour cell lines and viruses from contamination with the virus (ADAMS, ROWSON, and SALAMAN, 1961; NOTKINS, BERRY, MOLONEY, and GREENFIELD, 1962). If a contaminated tumour cell suspension is injected into newborn rats, the cells will survive for some time and the LDV will have disappeared by the 8th or 10th day after injection. The tumour cells can then be transplanted back into virus-free mice.

CRISPENS (1963b and d) reported attempts to isolate LDV from four human tumours, a mammary carcinoma, a leiomyosarcoma of stomach, a transitional cell kidney carcinoma and a melanoma of the choroid, but without success.

## C. Tissue Culture

The LDV replicates in cultures of various mouse tissues but the conditions necessary appear to be critical, and the virus is easily lost from a culture although the cells appear normal and other viruses may continue to replicate. It is therefore quite easy to free murine viruses which will replicate in tissue cultures from contamination with LDV. The Moloney leukaemia virus was freed from LDV by passage in mouse embryo tissue culture before the latter virus was known (ADAMS, ROWSON, and SALAMAN, 1961).

YAFFE (1962a and b) was the first to report the propagation of LDV in murine tissue cultures. He used cultures of embryo tissue and as there was no cytopathic

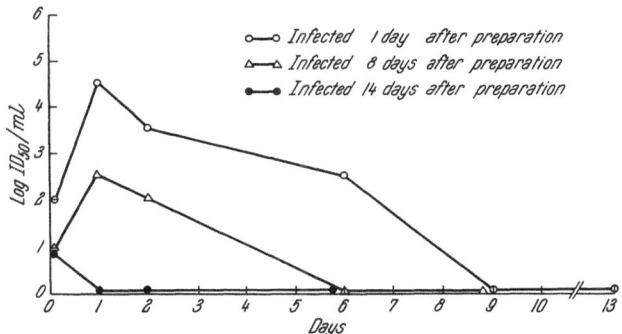

Fig. 32. Susceptibility of primary mouse embryo cultures to LDV infection. Titres of supernatant fluids of cultures infected on the 1st, 8th, and 14th day after preparation. (From EVANS and SALAMAN, 1965)

effect of the virus on the cells, the virus titre in the medium had to be titrated by injection into mice. YAFFE was able to propagate the virus indefinitely in primary mouse embryo tissue cultures by transferring medium every few days to new primary cultures. When infected cultures were trypsinized and replated, the virus was lost after the second passage and cultures in which the virus had died out could not be reinfected. That this was due to some change in the cultures on ageing and not to the action of the virus was shown by the fact that secondary and tertiary cultures, unexposed to the virus, were resistant to infection and could not be used successfully to replicate the virus. Figure 32 (EVANS, 1964; EVANS and SALAMAN, 1965) shows the LDV titre in mouse embryo cell cultures infected 1, 8, or 14 days after preparation. The infectivity is lost from the 14 day culture after 24 hours but infectivity is present for over a week in the youngest culture. However, even using freshly trypsinized primary embryo cultures, EVANS and SALAMAN (1965) were unable to maintain LDV in serial passage by either daily or twice weekly transfer. They compared cultures of mouse embryo liver and embryo-spleen, but though infectivity was maintained for longer than in whole embryo cultures, it was lost after 16 days. Using peritoneal macrophage cultures they were able to maintain infectivity for 22 days which was as long as the cultures would survive. By twice weekly passage into fresh macrophage cultures they were able to maintain the virus without loss of titre for 80 days.

Other workers have been more successful with mouse embryo cultures. ANDERSON and his colleagues (ANDERSON, RILEY, WADE, and MOORE, 1965; ANDERSON, RILEY, FITZMAURICE, LOVELESS, WADE, and MOORE, 1966) reported long periods of virus replication in primary cultures. In one experiment viral infectivity was still present after 119 days in culture. PLAGEMANN and SWIM (1966a) found that cultures produced virus until they had been subcultured 2 or 3 times which in the case of mouse embryo cultures was 2 to 3 weeks. Using adult mouse tissues the cultures grew more slowly, the interval between subcultures was therefore longer and viral infectivity persisted much longer. In one experiment a culture of adult lung cells continued to produce virus until the cells began to degenerate after 150 days in culture.

In contrast to these results, GEORGII and LENZ (1964) found that viral infectivity could be maintained in mouse embryo cultures for a maximum of 14 days, and DU BUY and JOHNSON (1966) observed a gradual decrease in virus titre over the course of 3 days. Both found that viral infectivity persisted longer in embryo cell cultures than in control tubes containing only tissue culture medium, but they obtained no definite evidence of viral replication in mouse embryo cell culture.

Of the many variations between the different reports, the factors of most importance in successful replication of LDV appear to be the tissue culture medium and the conditions of culture. The strain of mouse cells used seems to have little effect. DU BUY and JOHNSON (1968) compared macrophages from 3 strains, G.P., CDF and C57B6, and found no difference between them. They were able to maintain the virus by alternate passage in C57B6 and CDF cells, thus showing that virus released from one strain of cell could readily infect another. In their first experiment on the replication of LDV in macrophage cultures DU BUY and JOHNSON (1966) were unable to maintain the virus on serial passage. However, when they maintained the pH of the tissue culture medium more carefully the cultures continued to produce virus for at least 21 days and the virus could be maintained by serial passage to fresh cultures (DU BUY and JOHNSON, 1968). EVANS (1967) found that by replacing the lamb serum he had used in his earlier work (EVANS and SALAMAN, 1965) by calf serum he obtained very much prolonged virus replication in mouse embryo tissue cultures. He was able to maintain infection with LDV by twice weekly passage in primary mouse embryo tissue cultures and even to infect secondary cultures.

Although there are many reports that cultures from certain tissues or of certain cell types gave better results than others, there is no consensus of opinion and the conclusion must be that the nature of the cells in which LDV replicates is not at present clear. EVANS (1967) found that embryonic tissue was in general better than adult tissue for LDV replication, but whether this was due to cellular differentiation or to the loss of a highly susceptible cell type was not evident. The proportion of fibroblastic cells and phagocytic cells, which EVANS identified by their ability to take up zymosan, varied at different stages in the life of the primary embryo cultures, but this did not appear to affect virus production in the culture. The absence of epithelial cells in the older cultures which had disintegrated and regrown on the glass and which continued to produce virus, indicated that these cells were not necessary for viral replication. The role of lymphocytes in LDV replication in cultures of peritoneal cells was investigated by EVANS (1970). He used cultures with different proportions of macrophages and lymphocytes and found that virus replication was best in pure macrophage cultures. Pure lymphocyte cultures produced very little if any new virus.

A factor which may be of importance in preparing primary cultures suitable for LDV replication and in causing the loss of viral infectivity on preparation of secondary cultures is the strength of trypsin used. The virus is not inactivated by treatment with trypsin (0.2 mg per ml for 1 hour at 37° C) (DU BUY and JOHNSON, 1966), but certain cells or cell receptors may be. FRANTSI and GREGORY (1969) found that mouse embryo liver cell cultures prepared with 0.025 per cent trypsin were very much better for LDV replication than those prepared using 0.25 per cent trypsin. They were of the opinion that the stronger enzyme solution destroyed or altered cells which were particularly suitable for virus replication. In the cultures prepared with dilute trypsin, from 50 to 90 per cent of the cells showed a loss of cytoplasmic extensions, which were typical of those sensitive cells, within 6 to 8 hours after infection. By 14 hours, many of the cells had rounded up and had a deeply granular appearance. The virus titre in the medium started to rise two hours after infection and reached a peak by four hours after which it fell slowly. The LDH activity in the infected cultures was increased as compared to non-infected cultures from four hours after infection. FRANTSI and GREGORY (1969) are the only workers to have observed a cytopathic effect and an increased level of LDH activity in cultures infected with LDV. All the other reports (PLAGEMANN, WATANABE, and SWIM, 1962; GEORGII, LENZ, and ZOBEL, 1964; ANDERSON, RILEY, FITZMAURICE, LOVELESS, WADE, and MOORE, 1966; DU BUY and JOHNSON, 1966; NOTKINS, 1971a; YAMAZAKI and NOTKINS, (1973) agree in observing no cytopathic effect or increase of LDH activity in the medium of tissue cultures infected with LDV. The failure of the virus to cause any alteration in the LDH production of infected cells is not surprising as the bulk, if not all, of the increase in plasma LDH activity caused by the virus appears to be due to blockade of the reticuloendothelial system and not to increased enzyme production by the infected cells (see p. 65).

The lack of an obvious cytopathic effect in virus producing cultures is compatible with the prolonged virus production which occurs in cultures under ideal conditions, and with the observation that most of the virus infectivity is in the medium. One explanation for this is that the complete infective virus is formed at the cell surface and released into the medium without cell destruction. Alternatively, the proportion of cells in the culture which are producing virus may be very small. The observation that infection with LDV does not affect the rate of nucleic acid or protein synthesis in mixed cell cultures of spleen and lung cells (PLAGEMANN and SWIM, 1966a) does not help to decide between these two alternatives. However, OLDSTONE, YAMAZAKI, NIWA, and NOTKINS (1974) using immunofluorescent and infectious centre assays to estimate the proportion of cells producing virus in primary mouse embryo cell cultures infected with LDV found that only a small proportion were producing virus. The infectious centre experiments indicated that only 0.45 per cent of cells were virus producers 24 hours after infection. In the immunofluorescence studies, using an anti-LDV immunoglobulin, 2.2 per cent of cells stained at 24 hours, but at 48 hours only 0.3 per cent stained. It therefore seems likely that in cell cultures only a very few cells yield virus and even if these cells are destroyed they would not make an observable cytopathic effect.

Established tissue culture lines of mouse cells (mouse embryo strain 1, mouse lung strain 1, mouse kidney strain 33, and strain L mouse cells) appear unable to support LDV replication (PLAGEMANN and SWIM, 1966a), despite an earlier report that extracts of LDV inoculated L cells caused a significant rise in plasma LDH on injection into mice (GEORGII, JÄGER, KROTH, and BAYERLE, 1962). Other tissue culture cell systems which have been found not to support LDV replication are: HeLa, rhesus monkey kidney, rat peritoneal macrophages (PLAGEMANN and SWIM, 1966a; EVANS and SALAMAN, 1965; EVANS, 1964), suckling hamster kidney cells (TENNANT and WARD, 1962), and murine tumour cells from a number of transplantable tumours (YAFFE, 1962a and b; PLAGEMANN, GREGORY, SWIM, and CHAN, 1963; PLAGEMANN and SWIM, 1966a).

NOTKINS (1971a) and YAMAZAKI and NOTKINS (1973) were unable to demonstrate the presence of interferon activity in primary mouse embryo cells in which LDV was replicating, but if the cultures were incubated overnight with mouse interferon before infection with LDV the virus titre 24 hours later was depressed by over 99 per cent as compared with that in similar cultures not pretreated with interferon. DU BUY, BARON, UHLENDORF, and JOHNSON (1973) were unable to demonstrate interferon in unstimulated mouse macrophage cultures infected with LDV. Thus, in tissue cultures LDV appears to be a poor inducer of interferon but quite sensitive to its action. The possibility that small amounts of interferon, not detected by standard techniques, are formed in LDV infected tissue cultures and limit viral replication has been tested by treating the cultures with actinomycin D, which blocks interferon production, or any DNA-dependent synthesis of protein inhibitors. DU BUY and JOHNSON (1970) used mouse macrophage cultures and added actinomycin D 30 minutes before the LDV (1 or 3 µg per Leighton tube) and maintained the same concentration during virus replication. The lower concentration of actinomycin D only slightly reduced the concentration of virus in the medium at 8 hours after infection. The higher concentration reduced the virus titre from $10^{6.7}$ to $10^{5.5}$ $ID_{50}$/ml but the cells were noticeably more rounded up than in the control cultures. EVANS (1969 and 1970) also found that actinomycin D did not increase or prolong LDV replication in mouse peritoneal macrophage cultures, but there is one report (NOTKINS, 1971a) that LDV replication in primary mouse embryo cultures is inhibited by actinomycin D. NOTKINS (1971a) treated his cultures with actinomycin D for one hour before infection with LDV and found that as little as 0.125 µg/ml would reduce the yield of LDV by 98 per cent. These results give no support to the idea that interferon is cutting short LDV replication in tissue cultures and although actinomycin D may reduce the yield of LDV under certain conditions there must be some doubt as to whether or not a DNA-dependent RNA step is involved in LDV replication. To determine if DNA synthesis was required for LDV replication, YAMAZAKI and NOTKINS (1973) treated primary mouse embryo cultures with cytosine-β-D arabinofuranoside ($10^{-4}$ M) prior to infection and found that although DNA synthesis was inhibited by 60 per cent, LDV replication was not appreciably affected. Similarly, 5-fluorodeoxyuridine did not inhibit LDV replication. These results would not indicate the presence of an RNA-dependent DNA polymerase and NOTKINS (1971a) reports that one was not found in his virus preparations.

# VI. Pathogenesis

## A. Plasma Enzymes

Changes in the chemical composition of the blood may provide a sensitive index of the course of many diseases. Of the various normal and abnormal blood constituents, enzymes have proved of particular value to chemical pathologists since the high measurable activity associated with minute quantities of enzyme protein mean that small changes in their concentration can be detected with great sensitivity. However, for many years the only serum enzymes to be studied were acid and alkaline phosphatases, which were reported to alter in activity in bone and liver disease (ROBERTS, 1930, 1933). Over the subsequent twenty years, methods for the study of several other serum enzymes such as cholinesterases, lipase, amylase and aldolase were developed—see reviews by KING (1959) and WILKINSON (1962)—but it was not until interest in the so-called metabolic enzymes (lactate dehydrogenase, aspartate transaminase, alanine transaminase, and isocitrate dehydrogenase) intensified in the 1950's that the subject of serum enzymology suddenly attracted universal attention. Previously, increases in enzyme activity which had been reported were thought to result from simple obstruction of the normal secretory mechanisms, as for example the rise in alkaline phosphatase in liver disease involving obstruction of the bile ducts. The measurement of transaminase or lactate dehydrogenase activities in serum was considered, on the other hand, to provide an index of cell damage, and numerous reports appeared claiming the specificity of one enzyme rise or another for various disease conditions (see Table 10).

HILL and LEVI (1954) first reported that lactate dehydrogenase activity was increased in the serum of patients with neoplastic disease, and with the development of a satisfactory assay method for lactate dehydrogenase activity in blood (WRÓBLEWSKI and LADUE, 1955), mice bearing experimental tumours were found to have elevated plasma lactate dehydrogenase levels (HILL and JORDAN, 1957; HSIEH, SUNTZEFF, and COWDRY, 1956; JACOBSON and NISHIO, 1963; MANSO, SUGIURA, and WRÓBLEWSKI, 1958; FRIEND and WRÓBLEWSKI, 1956). It was during a study of the relationship between plasma LDH activity and tumour growth (RILEY and WRÓBLEWSKI, 1960) that LDV was discovered. When mice were implanted subcutaneously with Ehrlich carcinoma cells, five phases were observed in the alteration of LDH activity in the blood plasma (Fig. 1). Following tumour implantation there was a latent period of one to three days (Phase 1) which was followed by a rapid increase in enzyme activity from the normal levels

Table 10. *Serum Enzyme Activities Increased in Association with Certain Disease Conditions in Man*

| Serum enzymes | Disease | Reference |
|---|---|---|
| Alanine transaminase[a] | Liver disease | WRÓBLEWSKI and LA DUE (1956) |
| Aldolase | Muscular dystrophy | DREYFUS, SCHAPIRA and SCHAPIRA (1958) |
| Alkaline phosphatase | Osteoblastic disease<br>Jaundice | ROBERTS (1930)<br>ROBERTS (1933)<br>GUTMAN (1959) |
| Aspartate transaminase[b] | Myocardial infarction | KARMEN, WRÓBLEWSKI and LA DUE (1955) |
| | Hepatitis | WRÓBLEWSKI, JERVIS and LA DUE (1956) |
| γ-Glutamyl transpeptidase | Pancreatic or hepato-biliary disease | RUTENBURG, GOLDBERG and PINEDA (1963) |
| 2-Hydroxybutyrate dehydrogenase[c] | Myocardial infection | ELLIOT, JEPSON and WILKINSON (1962) |
| | Megaloblastic anaemia | ELLIOTT and WILKINSON (1963) |
| Isocitrate dehydrogenase | Viral hepatitis | WOLFSON, SPENCER, STERKEL and WILLIAMS-ASHMAN (1958) |
| Leucine aminopeptidase | Hepatobiliary disease | MERICAS, ANAGNOSTOU, HADZIYANNIS and KAKARI (1964) |
| Lactate dehydrogenase (Total) | Myocardial infarction<br>Neoplasia, Lymphoma<br>Breast<br>Gastrointestinal<br>Megaloblastic and Sickle cell anaemia | WRÓBLEWSKI (1959)<br>BIERMAN, HILL, REINHARDT and EMORY (1957)<br>ROSE, WEST and ZIMMERMAN (1961)<br>SCHWARTZ, WEST, WALSH and ZIMMERMAN (1962)<br>ZIMMERMAN, WEST and HELLER (1958) |
| Lactate dehydrogenase (H4 isoenzyme) | Myocardial infarction | VAN DER HELM, ZONDAG, HARTOG and VAN DER KOOI (1962)<br>BELL (1963) |
| Ornithine carbamyl transferase | Viral hepatitis | REICHARD (1961) |
| Phosphocreatine kinase | Muscular dystrophy | DREYFUS, SCHAPIRA and DEMOS (1960) |
| Sorbitol dehydrogenase | Parenchymal liver injury | ASADA and GALAMBOS (1963) |
| Triose-phosphate isomerase | Viral hepatitis | GIUSTI and PICCININO (1963) |

[a] Also known as glutamic-pyruvate transaminase.

[b] Also known as glutamic-oxaloacetic transaminase.

[c] Mainly measures LDH-4 isoenzyme.

Table 11. *The Effect of a Number of Viruses on Plasma Enzyme Activities in Recipient Mice*

| Virus inoculation | Days after inoculation | LDH (IU×10⁻²) | PGI (IU×10²) | AST (IU) | ALT (IU) | AlkP (IU×10⁻²) |
|---|---|---|---|---|---|---|
| Controls | Uninoculated | 2.08±0.16 (45)ᵃ 0.80−5.20ᵇ | 1.32±0.13 (43) 0−3.1ᵇ | 43±3.0 (39) 13−119ᵇ | 15±1.5 (33) 0−34ᵇ | 1.40±0.11 (41) 0.13−3.18ᵇ |
| Friend leukaemia | 2 | 1.70±0.17 (8) | 1.29±0.10 (8) | 22±4.4 (8) | 10±4.2 (8) | 1.10±0.09 (8) |
| | 4 | 1.35±0.30 (8) | 0.91±0.07 (7) | 35±4.0 (7) | 20±3.9 (7) | 1.19±0.07 (7) |
| | 7 | 1.15±0.08 (8) | 0.94±0.05 (8) | 35±2.8 (7) | 29±1.9 (8) | 0.96±0.07 (8) |
| | 10 | 1.08±0.06 (8) | 0.70±0.04 (8) | 32±3.1 (6) | 25±2.2 (6) | 0.79±0.06 (8) |
| Moloney leukaemia | 2 | 1.77±0.23 (6) | 1.23±0.17 (6) | 43±5.6 (6) | 14±2.3 (5) | 1.14±0.10 (5) |
| | 4 | 2.50±0.18 (6) | 1.37±0.14 (6) | 35±2.6 (5) | 11±1.7 (6) | 0.98±0.18 (6) |
| | 7 | 2.90±0.43 (6) | 1.30±0.07 (6) | 49±6.4 (5) | 11±2.9 (5) | 1.10±0.16 (6) |
| | 10 | 1.10±0.11 (6) | 0.80±0.08 (6) | 32±2.9 (6) | 12±1.8 (6) | 1.02±0.16 (6) |
| Polyoma | 2 | 4.20±0.82 (6) | 1.65±0.54 (6) | 70±11.2 (6) | 6±0 (5) | 0.93±0.08 (4) |
| | 4 | 2.27±0.52 (6) | 1.87±0.34 (6) | 50±5.1 (4) | 19±3.2 (5) | 0.85±0.11 (4) |
| | 7 | 3.40±0.67 (6) | — | 63±14.5 (6) | 12±1.8 (6) | 0.80 (3) |
| | 10 | 1.07±0.10 (6) | 2.32±0.46 (6) | 43±3.1 (5) | 10±4.1 (5) | 0.88±0.23 (4) |
| Vaccinia | 2 | 3.97±0.55 (6) | 2.48±0.82 (6) | 56±11.0 (5) | 13±1.4 (5) | 0.83±0.16 (4) |
| | 4 | 2.77±0.58 (6) | 1.25±0.29 (6) | 52±5.0 (6) | 11±1.7 (4) | 1.15±0.21 (4) |
| | 7 | 2.57±0.55 (6) | 0.65±0.24 (6) | 62±11.3 (6) | 11±3.6 (6) | 1.90 (2) |
| | 10 | 3.30±0.35 (6) | 3.73±0.27 (6) | 48±5.0 (6) | 11±3.2 (5) | 1.00±0.09 (5) |
| Influenza A | 2 | 3.20±0.63 (6) | 0.78±0.07 (6) | 55±6.3 (6) | 6±2.2 (6) | 0.84±0.09 (5) |
| | 4 | 1.43±0.22 (6) | 0.65±0.25 (6) | 54±7.2 (6) | 16±1.5 (6) | 1.50±0.16 (6) |
| | 7 | 2.90±0.29 (4) | — | 47 (3) | 11 (3) | 2.35±0.67 (4) |
| | 10 | 1.24±0.30 (5) | 3.06±0.50 (5) | 50±11.9 (5) | 12±3.3 (5) | 0.38±0.06 (5) |
| LCM | 2 | 2.50±0.38 (6) | 0.45±0.21 (6) | 51±9.7 (5) | 33±15 (6) | 1.98±0.35 (4) |
| | 4 | 3.53±0.54 (6) | 2.47±0.36 (6) | 55±8.3 (6) | | 1.68±0.23 (4) |
| | 7 | 3.07 (3) | 2.50 (3) | 69 (3) | 14 (3) | 0.85 (2) |
| | 10 | — | — | — | — | — |

ᵃ Results expressed as means ± standard error of mean. Number of animals given in parentheses.
ᵇ Range.

of 400 to 600 international units to between 2,000 and 6,000 units (Phase 2). At this time, tumour growth was still not measurable, and it was found that plasma LDH activity remained at a constant plateau level for several days (Phase 3). When growth of tumour mass became detectable, a second rapid rise in LDH activity occurred (Phase 4), with maximum levels of 40,000 units being observed. Finally, there was a fall in plasma LDH activity (Phase 5) just prior to the death of the animal. Mice treated with orthophenylenediamine, which caused regression of the tumour, were found to have lowered plasma LDH activity, but although some mice remained free of the tumour for several months, their plasma LDH level never returned completely to normal but remained at 4,000 to 6,000 units (RILEY and WRÓBLEWSKI, 1960). It was subsequently shown that the early tenfold rise in plasma LDH activity occurring within the first four days after tumour implantation could also be obtained if plasma from tumour-bearing mice were used as inoculum, and moreover that this capacity to increase plasma LDH activity was serially transmissible (RILEY, LILLY, HUERTO, and BARDELL, 1960). These studies established the viral nature of the early increase in plasma LDH activity, and made way for extensive studies on the nature of plasma enzyme elevation by this virus.

## B. Plasma Enzyme Levels in LDV Infected Mice

Figure 4 shows the changes in plasma LDH activity occurring in the blood of mice following infection with LDV. From 24 to 72 hours following infection, enzyme activity rises approximately tenfold and remains elevated for at least one year, probably throughout the lifespan of the animal (ROWSON, ADAMS and SALAMAN, 1963; GEORGII, 1962). Various workers have demonstrated that the rate at which plasma LDH activity rises following infection is to some extent dependent on the magnitude of the infecting dose (NOTKINS and SHOCHAT, 1963; RILEY, 1968b) (Fig. 5). The higher the infective dose, at least over the range 10 $ID_{50}$ to $10^8$ $ID_{50}$, the more rapid is the initial increase in enzyme activity. However, from 96 hours after infection, plasma LDH levels are similar in all mice whatever the initial dose injected (NOTKINS and SHOCHAT, 1963). Figure 4 shows that the appearance of virus in the circulation precedes the increase in plasma LDH activity in individual

Table 12. *Changes in Activity of Plasma Enzymes*

| Authors | Enzymes | | |
|---|---|---|---|
| | LDH | ICD | MDH |
| PLAGEMANN, WATANABE and SWIM, 1962 | +++[a] | +++ | ++ |
| NOTKINS, GREENFIELD, MARSHALL and BANE, 1963 | +++ | +++ | ++ |
| MAHY, ROWSON, SALAMAN and PARR, 1964 | +++ | NS | NS |

[a] + Significant elevation.
[b] − No change.
[c] NS Enzyme not studied.

mice, so that there is no obvious correlation between the two parameters. Nevertheless, the fact that the rate of increase in plasma LDH activity does depend on the size of the virus inoculum supports the notion that there is a close link between the two parameters.

RILEY (1968b) has published extensive studies in which the normal distribution of plasma LDH activities in uninfected and LDV infected mice were determined. These show that even when very large populations of mice are sampled, there is no overlap between the highest plasma LDH activities in normal uninfected mice and the lowest activities which can be observed in infected mice. The plasma LDH activities of normal mice are in fact very constant, and though it has been reported that there are minor strain-to-strain variations in mean LDH level (CRISPENS, 1963c), these have not been found by others (RILEY, 1968b). The sex of mice does not influence plasma LDH activity, but age has some effect, as very young animals, from birth to approximately three weeks, have higher LDH levels than mice which have reached sexual maturity (RILEY, 1968b).

Soon after the viral nature of the LDH-elevating agent had been established, a report appeared in which it was suggested that increases in plasma LDH activity were in no way confined to infections with LDV, but that mice infected with other viruses, namely Friend, polyoma, Newcastle disease, vaccinia and Columbia SK (encephalomyocarditis) viruses all possessed raised serum LDH levels (WENNER, MILLIAN, MIRAND, and GRACE, 1962). The increased enzyme activity was attributed to erythrocyte destruction occurring in the blood of infected mice, with consequent release of LDH into the serum. In an attempt to confirm these results, MAHY and his colleagues (MAHY, PARR, and ROWSON, 1963b; MAHY, ROWSON, SALAMAN, and PARR, 1964) examined the levels of plasma LDH, as well as a number of other enzymes, in mice infected with Friend, Moloney mouse leukaemia viruses, polyoma, vaccinia, influenza A, lymphocytic choriomeningitis, and encephalomyocarditis viruses (Table 11). Provided the virus preparations were free from contamination with LDV (see above) none of these viruses, except encephalomyocarditis virus, caused any significant change in plasma enzyme levels. It was further shown that the enzyme changes induced by encephalomyocarditis virus, which caused extensive pathological changes and death within three days in infected mice, were of a

*after LDV Infection as Studied by Various Workers*

| | Enzymes | | | | | | | | |
|------|------|------|------|------|------|------|------|------|------|
| GR | PHI | GOT | ALD | GPD | G-6PD | AKP | ACP | GPT | LAP |
| ++ | ++ | ++ | — b | — | — | — | — | — | — |
| NS c | ++ | ++ | — | NS | NS | — | NS | NS | NS |
| NS | +++ | ++ | — | NS | NS | — | — | + | NS |

LDH = Lactate dehydrogenase; ICD = Isocitrate dehydrogenase; MDH = Malate dehydrogenase; GR = Glutathione reductase; PHI = Phosphohexose isomerase; GOT = Glutamic-oxaloacetic transaminase; ALD = Aldolase; GPD = Alpha-glycerophosphate dehydrogenase; G-6PD = Glucose-6-phosphate dehydrogenase; AKP = Alkaline phosphatase; ACP = Acid phosphatase; GPT = Glutamic-pyruvic transaminase; LAP = Leucine aminopeptidase.

different type to those induced by LDV (Fig. 6), and were directly related to the severity of tissue damage. Thus, it seems reasonable to conclude that LDV retains a unique position in causing permanently raised LDH levels in the plasma of infected mice without significant tissue damage.

Although the original recognition of LDV was due to its ability to increase the plasma LDH level of infected mice, it soon became evident that a number of other plasma enzymes were also affected (MAHY, PARR, and ROWSON, 1963; NOTKINS, GREENFIELD, MARSHALL, and BANE, 1963; BAYERLE, GEORGII, and RICHARD, 1962; NOTKINS, 1963b; PLAGEMANN, WATANABE, and SWIM, 1962; MAHY, ROWSON, SALAMAN, and PARR, 1964). Table 12 lists the reported changes in plasma activity of various enzymes as studied by different workers. The most striking increases are observed in LDH, isocitrate dehydrogenase, and phosphohexose isomerase, all of which increase up to tenfold after infection. A number of other enzymes increase from two-to-four-fold and these include malate dehydrogenase, aspartate transaminase (also known as glutamic-oxaloacetic transaminase), glutathione reductase and alanine transaminase (also known as glutamic pyruvic transaminase). Finally, no significant changes are observed following infection, in the plasma activities of aldolase, acid and alkaline phosphatase, leucine aminopeptidase, alpha-glycerophosphate dehydrogenase, or glucose-6-phosphate dehydrogenase.

The enzymes which are found to increase in activity in LDV infected mice cannot be grouped together on any obvious basis such as function, tissue localization, or molecular size, although all are probably of cytoplasmic origin (PLAGEMANN, WATANABE, and SWIM. 1962), However, several of those enzymes which occur in the cytoplasmic cell fraction are not altered by LDV infection.

## C. Origin of Raised Plasma Enzyme Activities

### 1. Increased Tissue Breakdown

The plasma enzyme activities measured in normal animals are believed to represent breakdown products of effected cells. The observed activity presumably represents a balance between the rate at which enzyme proteins enter the plasma and the rate at which they are removed or become inactivated. In some pathological conditions, increases in enzyme activity in plasma can be ascribed to damage occurring in a particular cell type (WILKINSON, 1962), and many investigators therefore attempted to relate the particular pattern of raised plasma enzyme activities found in LDV infection to a tissue in which the virus was purported to replicate. A possible clue was provided by the observation that only one of the five naturally occurring isoenzymes of LDH found in mouse plasma was significantly elevated following LDV infection (PLAGEMANN, GREGORY, SWIM, and CHAN, 1963; WARNOCK, 1964). This isoenzyme (LDH-V), the slowest migrating one, was found to occur in high concentration in mouse liver, spleen and erythrocytes, and these organs were therefore implicated as possible sites of virus replication. The moderate splenomegaly which was occasionally found in infected mice (RILEY, 1963b; POPE, 1963) coupled with a report that mouse spleen cells grown *in vitro* would support the replication of LDV (PLAGEMANN and SWIM, 1962), prompted a more careful examination of the role of the spleen in infected mice. However, no differences were found in plasma LDH level or plasma virus titre between uninoculated intact and splenectomized mice, or between intact and splenectomized mice up to 16 days after LDV inoculation (Fig. 33) (ROWSON, MAHY, and EVANS, 1963; RILEY, 1963c).

No comparable studies have been reported concerning the role of the liver in pathogenesis, but in an attempt to demonstrate increased release of LDH from spleen or liver cells derived from LDV infected mice, ROWSON, MAHY, and EVANS (1963) made trypsinized suspensions from adult spleen and liver and cultured these for up to six days at 37° C. The LDH activity of the culture fluids was determined at intervals, but no significant differences were recorded in cultures prepared

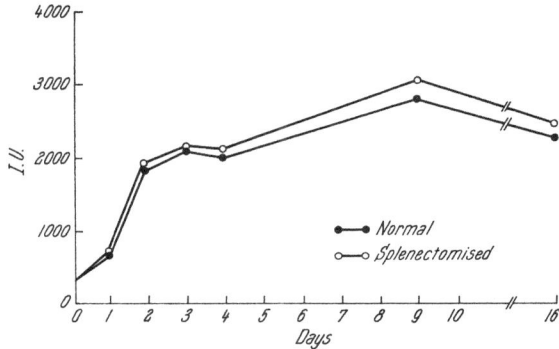

Fig. 33. Plasma LDH activity following LDV infection in normal and splenectomized mice

from infected mice compared to those prepared from normal mice of the same age and strain. No histological changes are demonstrable by light or electron microscopy in the liver, so it would seem unlikely that there can be much tissue damage with release of LDH.

The possibility that the increase in plasma LDH might be due to erythrocyte destruction was studied by RILEY (1963d). He observed a slight depression in haematocrit, red blood cell count, and total haemoglobin in infected mice, and this was also found by BAILEY, STEARMAN, and CLOUGH (1963). A much more severe anaemia was observed when the virus was inoculated into splenectomized or tumour-bearing mice (RILEY, 1964; RILEY, HUERTO, LOVELESS, BARDELL, FITZMAURICE, and FORMAN, 1963), but in this case the anaemia was not due to LDV but to the presence of a Bartonella-like organism, *Eperythrozoon coccoides* (RILEY, 1968b). When such an anaemia was observed in infected mice, there was a dramatic rise in plasma LDH activity, showing that erythrocyte destruction can certainly induce an elevation in the activity of this plasma enzyme. Indeed, it was suggested at this time that the presence of eperythrozoon infection contributed to the early rise in plasma LDH occurring after inoculation of mice with transplantable tumour cells (ARISON, CASSARO, and SHONK, 1963). Careful studies by RILEY's group (RILEY, 1964; RILEY, LOVELESS, and FITZMAURICE, 1964) established that most laboratory passages of eperythrozoon were already contaminated with LDV due to transfer in mice, and furthermore that eperythrozoon was present in some stocks of LDV. The eperythrozoon preparation was freed of LDV by passage in rats, in which the virus does not multiply, and the LDV was freed of eperythrozoon by treatment of infected mice with the arsenical drug 2-amino-4-arsenophenol hydrochloride (0.5 mg per mouse). When the two agents were injected separately into test mice they were found to have quite different effects on plasma LDH level. LDV induced a permanent rise in enzyme activity 48 hours after inoculation, whereas *Eperythrozoon coccoides* infection had a variable effect on plasma LDH activity, depending on the maximum titre attained during the infection and whether or not the host was splenectomized. By 10 to 14 days the enzyme activity had invariably returned to normal. LDV has a potentiating effect on the severity of the disease caused by *Eperythrozoon coccoides* (FITZMAURICE, RILEY, and SANTISTEBAN, 1972).

That erythrocyte destruction is not the cause of the increased plasma enzyme activities in LDV infected mice was established by BAILEY, CLOUGH, and STEARMAN (1964a). They measured the enzyme content of erythrocytes, and calculated that 4.1 per cent haemolysis was necessary to account for the observed increase in plasma LDH of infected mice. They found, however, that the malate dehydrogenase content of erythrocytes was double that of LDH, and should have resulted in a 2.5-fold increase in malate dehydrogenase in LDV infected mouse plasma: this was not observed (BAILEY, CLOUGH, and STEARMAN, 1964a). Similarly, the erythrocyte content of glutamic-oxaloacetic transaminase should have raised the plasma activity by 2.3-fold, but no such increase was observed. Thus, neither spleen, liver nor erythrocytes can be the sole origin of the raised plasma enzyme activities.

## 2. Increased Enzyme Synthesis

Since no evidence of tissue damage likely to be the cause of increased plasma enzyme activity could be found, several investigators examined the hypothesis that LDV stimulates *de novo* synthesis of certain enzymes which are then released into the plasma (PLAGEMANN, WATANABE, and SWIM, 1962; BAILEY, STEARMAN, and CLOUGH, 1963; WARNOCK, 1964; RILEY, FITZMAURICE, LOVELESS, KRYZAK, GALLAGHER, and SILER, 1965; RILEY, HUERTO, BARDELL, FITZMAURICE, and LOVELESS, 1963).

The most complete study was made by PLAGEMANN and SWIM (1962), who measured the activities of three enzymes, lactate dehydrogenase, isocitrate dehydrogenase and glutamic-pyruvate transaminase in the following tissues from normal and LDV infected mice: liver, kidney, heart, lung, skeletal muscle, spleen, erythrocytes and plasma. No increased enzyme activity was observed in any tissue from infected mice except plasma. BAILEY, STEARMAN, and CLOUGH (1963) measured LDH activities in all these tissues, and in brain, pancreas, submaxillary gland and thymus with the same negative results. WARNOCK (1964) made similar observations.

It should be pointed out that although the replication of some viruses, notably those containing DNA as genetic material (KEIR, 1968), is accompanied by synthesis of several new enzymes in infected cells, these are invariably associated with nucleic acid replication and not with cellular metabolic functions. It is not surprising, therefore, that LDV is no exception to this general rule. At least seven different enzyme activities increase in plasma of LDV infected mice, and it seems unlikely that the *de novo* synthesis of all seven could be increased in a specific way by the virus.

## 3. Changes in Enzyme Activity in Supernatants of Tissue Cultures Replicating LDV

Increases in the activity of LDH and aspartate transaminase have been observed in the medium of tissue cultures replicating a wide range of viruses including poliovirus (GEVAUDAN, GEVAUDAN, GAY, and ARNAUD, 1960) lymphocytic choriomeningitis virus (GEVAUDAN, GAY, and ARNAUD, 1961) echovirus type 12, Sendai virus (GILBERT, 1963) adenoviruses types 7 and 12 (GILBERT, 1963; LATNER, GARDNER, TURNER, and BROWN, 1964) and Semliki Forest virus (CASSELLS, 1973). In almost all cases where it has been studied, LDV was found to replicate in cell cultures *in vitro* without causing any cytopathic effect or increase in the LDH activity in the medium (GEORGII, THORN, and WRBA, 1966a; PLAGEMANN and SWIM, 1966a; DU BUY and JOHNSON, 1966; YAFFE, 1962a and b; ANDERSON, RILEY, FITZMAURICE, LOVELESS, WADE, and MOORE, 1966). There is a single report that in some circumstances LDV induces a cytopathic effect in mouse embryonic liver cell cultures, and in this case an increase in LDH activity of the culture medium is observed (FRANTSI and GREGORY, 1969). Therefore for LDV, as other viruses (GILBERT, 1963), enzyme release from tissue cultures does not occur unless accompanied by cellular injury. There is no evidence from these studies that LDV replication is associated with increased synthesis or production of LDH or other metabolic enzymes, or with an increase in cell membrane permeability resulting in leakage of enzyme from the host cells.

## 4. Impaired Enzyme Clearance from the Plasma of Infected Mice

### a) LDH Clearance in Normal and Infected Mice

There is now a considerable body of evidence to indicate that the principal cause of increased plasma enzyme activity in LDV-infected mice is an impairment of reticuloendothelial function resulting in a decreased rate of elimination of certain enzymes from the blood. The hypothesis that impaired 'clearance' (removal from the blood) of LDH and other enzymes might be responsible for the observed changes in activity following LDV infection was first put forward in 1964 by MAHY, ROWSON, SALAMAN, and PARR. It was argued that if LDV impaired the plasma enzyme clearance mechanism, both the enzyme rises in infected mice and the synergic increases observed with some enzymes during growth of tumours could readily be understood.

Earlier, WAKIM and FLEISHER (FLEISHER and WAKIM, 1963a and b; WAKIM and FLEISHER, 1963a and b) had reported that in dogs the rates of elimination of several different enzymes varied widely, but were characteristic for each enzyme protein. This suggested an explanation for the observation that only certain plasma enzymes were elevated by LDV, *i.e.* only those enzymes having similar rates of elimination might be influenced by infection.

Studies were made in several laboratories on the rates of elimination of exogenous LDH from plasma of normal and LDV-infected mice, which soon established that infection did indeed result in impaired LDH clearance (MAHY, 1964; NOTKINS and SCHEELE, 1964; BAILEY, CLOUGH, and STEARMAN, 1964b; CLOUGH and BAILEY, 1965; NOTKINS, 1965b; RILEY, LOVELESS, FITZMAURICE, and SILER, 1965; MAHY, ROWSON, and PARR, 1965). At the time these experiments were initiated, little was known of the factors determining clearance of enzymes from the blood in mice. In dogs, two distinct phases, fast then slow, of enzyme elimination were usually observed and in some cases a third rapid phase was noted (FLEISHER and WAKIM, 1963a and b). In no case could the elimination of enzyme be accounted for by urinary excretion, and splenectomy had no effect on clearance rates. It was also established that in dogs, clearance was a genuine removal of enzyme protein from the blood, and not a loss of enzyme activity as for example due to presence of inhibitors of the active site (WAKIM and FLEISHER, 1963a and b).

This is important, since peptides capable of inhibiting both the M and H subunits of human or rabbit muscle LDH (WILSON, KAPLAN, LEVINE, PESCE, REICHLIN, and ALLISON, 1964; SALTHE, CHILSON and KAPLAN, 1965) have been isolated from human urine (WACKER and SCHOENENBERGER, 1966). Studies made in pigs (MASSARRAT, 1965), rabbits (SCHAPIRA, DREYFUS, and SCHAPIRA, 1962) sheep (BOYD, 1967a and b) and mice (MAHY and WACHSMUTH, 1973), also established that enzyme clearance after intravenous injection was directly correlated with removal of enzyme protein from the blood.

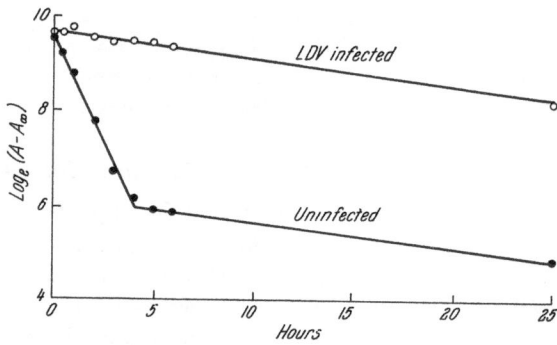

Fig. 34. Clearance of LDH from the plasma of an uninfected mouse, and a mouse which had been infected with LDV 10 days previously.
Each mouse was injected with 18,000 IU intravenously. (From MAHY, ROWSON, and PARR, 1967)

Early studies on the disappearance of LDH activity from mouse blood after intravenous injection of rabbit muscle-derived enzyme showed that in mice, as in dogs, the clearance rate was biphasic (Fig. 34). Normal, uninfected mice eliminated all injected LDH from the plasma within 24 hours, and the disappearance rates could be analysed graphically by applying a biphasic exponential equation of the form:

$$A = a_1 e^{-\lambda_1 t} + a_2 e^{-\lambda_2 t} + A_\infty$$

where A represents the plasma activity at any time (t), $A_\infty$ represents the plasma activity of the steady state (prior to injection), and $a_1$, $a_2$, $\lambda_1$ and $\lambda_2$ are essential arbitrary constants. A plot of $\log_e (A—A_\infty)$ therefore yields two straight lines, with slopes corresponding to $\lambda_1$ and $\lambda_2$, slow and fast phases, respectively. In mice, as in dogs, there was occasionally a suggestion of a third, faster rate of clearance with constant $\lambda_3$, but this was not always observed (MAHY, 1964). It is not clear what the three rate constants represent; a three-compartment catenary model, similar to models derived from studies of plasma protein turnover (KEKKI and EISALO, 1964) was suggested by FLEISHER and WAKIM (1963a) in explanation of their experimental observations. In this (Fig. 35) there are three interconnecting

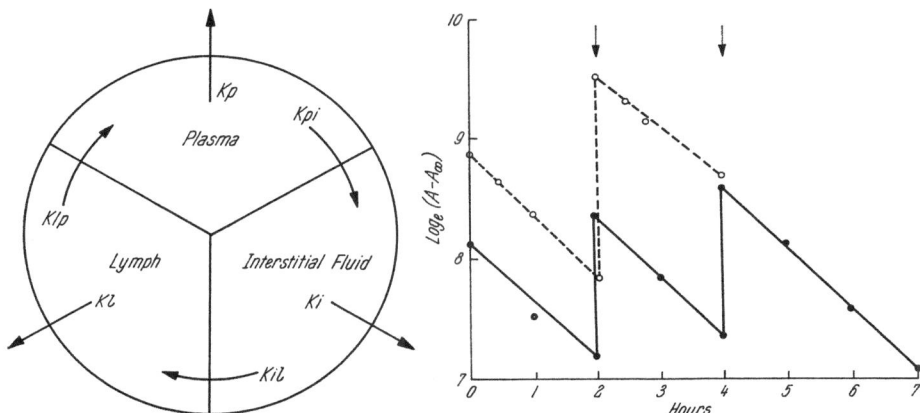

Fig. 35. A three-compartment catenary model. Enzyme is eliminated from the 3 interconnecting compartments. The observed rate constants $\lambda_1$, $\lambda_2$ and $\lambda_3$ describe the final rates of elimination which are related but not identical to the actual rate constants Kp, Ki and Kl

Fig. 36. Clearance of LDH from the plasma after intravenous injection of 3,000 (●———●) or 7,000 (○ − − − ○)IU, respectively, into groups of normal mice. Each point represents a mean value obtained from four mice. Arrows show reinjection times. (From MAHY, ROWSON, and PARR, 1967)

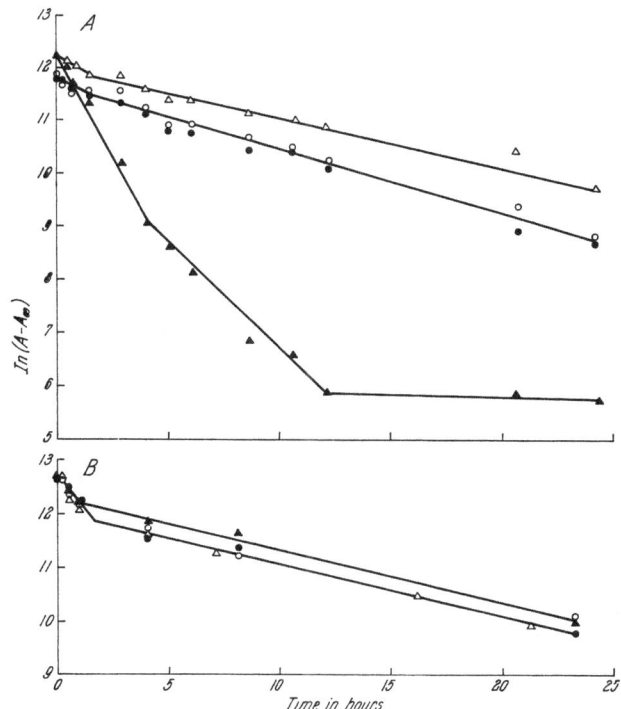

Fig. 37. Clearance of LDH isoenzymes I and V after intravenous injection into normal mice or mice infected 7 to 14 days previously with LDV.
Each mouse received 1.5 to $2.0 \times 10^5$ IU of either LDH-I or LDH-V isoenzyme
Each point represents the mean value obtained from two mice. In panel A the enzymes were as isolated. In panel B they were acetylated so as to remove the charge difference between them
●———● LDH-I in uninfected mice, ▲———▲ LDH-V in uninfected mice, ○———○ LDH-I in infected mice, △———△ LDH-V in infected mice

compartments, the plasma, lymph and interstitial fluid spaces, and elimination of enzyme is considered to occur in all three. The observed rate constants ($\lambda_1$, $\lambda_2$ and $\lambda_3$) describe the final rates of elimination, which are related, but not identical to the actual rate constants (Kp, Ki, Kl). This model provides one explanation for the experimental findings, but precise information as to the nature of the three compartments and their interrelationship is not available. Certainly it is practicable to analyse the clearance rates of enzymes injected into normal mice into only two phases, fast and slow.

When analysed in this way, it is found that in LDV-infected mice the fast clearance phase is either greatly reduced, or not present at all (MAHY, ROWSON, and PARR, 1967) (Fig. 34). Studies on the nature of the fast clearance phase of rabbit muscle LDH showed that it could not be blocked by repeated injections of enzyme at two and four hours after the initial dose (MAHY, ROWSON, and PARR, 1967) (Fig. 36). Later studies in which very high doses (up to 200,000 units) of mouse-derived LDH were injected into mice confirmed this earlier finding (Fig. 37) (MAHY and WACHSMUTH, 1973). Evidence was obtained, however, to suggest that injected enzyme is cleared at the fast rate only down to a critical plasma level, about 800 IU per litre, suggesting that the switch from fast to slow clearance involves some kind of threshold mechanism.

Studies on LDH clearance from normal mouse plasma were also made by BAILEY, CLOUGH, and STEARMAN (1964 a and b) and NOTKINS and SCHEELE (1964) but these authors did not attempt detailed analysis of their results. In some experiments, clearance was followed after intraperitoneal injections of LDH: this leads to a complex interaction where the plasma LDH level is changing due to influx from the peritoneal cavity as well as efflux from the blood. Nevertheless, in each case where it was studied, LDV infection decreased the apparent clearance of injected LDH (BAILEY, CLOUGH, and STEARMAN, 1964 b; MAHY, 1964; NOTKINS and SCHEELE, 1964; RILEY, LOVELESS, FITZMAURICE, and SILER, 1965).

RILEY, LOVELESS, FITZMAURICE, and SILER (1965) argued that it was best to ignore the early biphasic period of LDH clearance, on the grounds that secondary extra-vascular diffusion compartments were irrelevant to the long term clearance process. In so doing, they failed to demonstrate the absence of the fast clearance phase in LDV-infected mice. Since the virus affects the slow clearance phase only slightly, they concluded that the degree of LDH elevation observed in infected mouse plasma could not be entirely accounted for by impaired enzyme clearance (RILEY, LOVELESS, FITZMAURICE, and SILER, 1965; RILEY, 1968 b). It seems likely that in discarding the early plasma enzyme readings, these authors missed the essential observation that in LDV-infected mice the fast clearance phase is greatly reduced or absent. This can only be studied at high exogenous LDH inputs where the fast clearance mechanism is saturated with respect to enzyme. When the fast clearance phase is taken into account, the impairment in LDV-infected mice can wholly account for the observed rises in plasma LDH activity.

For example, in the analysis applied by RILEY, LOVELESS, FITZMAURICE, and SILER (1965) the enzyme level (E) at any time, (t), is given by:

$$(E—E\infty) = (Eo—E\infty)e^{-Ct}$$

in which the equilibrium level $E\infty = I/C$

where E is the activity at time t, $E\infty$ the steady state activity, I the rate of influx and C the clearance coefficient. The latter is calculated from

$$C = \frac{\log_e 2}{T\frac{1}{2}} = \frac{0.693}{T\frac{1}{2}}$$

where $T\frac{1}{2}$ is the time required to reduce the enzyme elevation level $(E - E\infty)$ by one half.

The rate of influx, I, is given by:

$$I = C \, E\infty$$

Whilst the absolute values of the clearance coefficient and influx rates are dependent on their true nature (model dependent) their ratios are not therefore:

$$\frac{I_1}{I_2} = \frac{C_1}{C_2} \times \frac{E\infty_1}{E\infty_2}$$

where $E\infty_2$ is the steady-state plasma activity of infected mice and $I_2$ the influx.

Applying this equation to an actual example (data are those used in MAHY, 1964, Table 1):

|  | Mean plasma LDH activity (4 mice) | Half-time of inject-ed LDH (hours) | Clearance Coefficient |
|---|---|---|---|
| Uninfected | 360 | 1.3±0.2 | 0.534 |
| Infected 3 days | 2000 | 8.0±1.0 | 0.087 |

$$\frac{I_1}{I_2} = \frac{0.534}{0.087} \times \frac{360}{2000} = \frac{192}{174} = 1.1$$

The enzyme influx is not increased, and if anything is less in the infected mice. Similar results were obtained on working out LDH half-times at different periods after infection.

Five isoenzymes of LDH can be separated by electrophoresis. These isoenzymes are tetramers composed of different proportions of two monomers. CAHN, KAPLAN, LEVINE, and ZWILLING (1962) called the monomers H and M, and the tetramers $H_4$, $H_3M$, $H_2M_2$, $H_1M_3$ and $M_4$ (LDH-I to LDH-V).

Studies by PLAGEMANN, GREGORY, SWIM, and CHAN (1963) and WARNOCK (1964) demonstrated that in plasma of LDV-infected mice the slowest migrating isoenzyme, LDH-V was greatly increased whereas the fastest migrating, LDH-I was not affected. It was therefore of interest to determine whether impaired clearance of intravenously injected LDH was specific for the LDH-V isoenzyme. Previous studies had employed rabbit muscle-derived enzyme (MAHY, 1964); this consisted primarily of LDH-V.

When the rates of clearance of LDH-I and LDH-V were measured in normal and LDV-infected mice, two conclusions were reached (MAHY and ROWSON, 1965). First, the clearance of LDH-I was very much slower than that of LDH-V in normal mice. Second, LDV-infection caused a dramatic decrease in clearance rate of LDH-V without significantly affecting that of LDH-I. In their experiments the LDH-I was derived from pig heart, and the LDH-V from rabbit muscle. The validity of comparing clearance rates of heterologous enzymes is not certain, but in subsequent experiments (MAHY and WACHSMUTH, unpublished) essentially the same results were obtained when homologous mouse-derived LDH isoenzymes were injected into mice. The difference in clearance rate between the two iso-enzymes appears to be a general phenomenon, since BOYD (1967a and b) obtained a similar result when measuring the disappearance of sheep-derived LDH-I and V isoenzymes from the plasma of normal sheep. For other enzymes, too, wide differences in clearance rates of isoenzymes have been reported, *e.g.* glutamic-oxaloacetic (aspartate) transaminase (FLEISHER and WAKIM, 1963b) and asparaginase (BROOME, 1965).

Further studies on the clearance rates of LDH isoenzymes in mice were made using all five types derived from pig tissue, (MAHY and WACHSMUTH, 1973; WACHSMUTH and KLINGMUELLER, 1973). The rate of clearance of each isoenzyme in

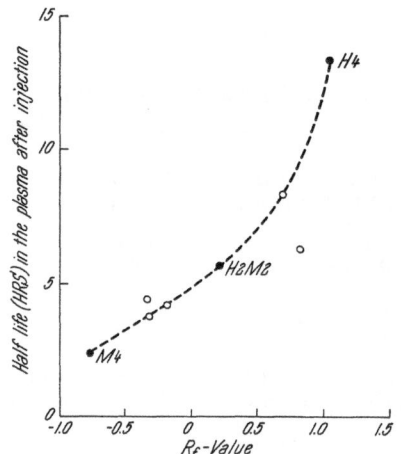

Fig. 38. Clearance rates of LDH isoenzymes from the plasma of normal mice. The half life of each isoenzyme (LDH-I, H4; LDH-III, H2M2 and LDH-V, M4) is plotted against electrophoretic mobility (●). Values for acetylated LDH isoenzymes with intermediate electrophoretic mobilities are also plotted (○)

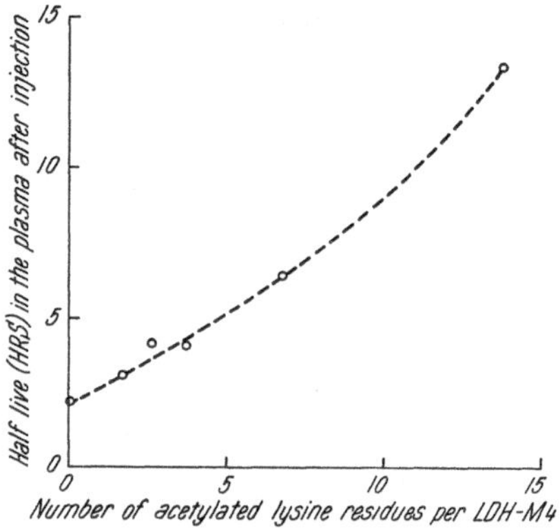

Fig. 39. Effect of acetylation of lysine residues in LDH-V (M4) upon the clearance rate from the plasma of normal mice

normal mice was directly correlated with the charge on the enzyme molecule, LDH-V being cleared at the fastest rate, and LDH-I at the slowest (Fig. 37, 38). The charge on LDH-V is contributed mainly by possession of twelve lysine residues in excess over LDH-I. When the LDH-V molecule was progressively acetylated to remove the lysine charge, the rate of clearance of the enzyme was correlated with the number of acetylated lysine residues (Fig. 39). When seven lysine residues were acetylated, the clearance rate of LDH-V became equal to that of LDH-I.

The results led to the conclusion that the charge on the LDH molecule is primarily responsible for the fast phase of enzyme clearance. This was confirmed using antibodies directed against the enzyme active site and specific for either LDH-I or LDH-V (WACHSMUTH, unpublished). LDH-V molecules which had been neutralized by acetylation of the lysine residues and were cleared at the slowest rate, as LDH-I, still reacted specifically with anti-LDH-V sera and were not neutralized by anti-LDH-I sera.

In mice infected with LDV, all isoenzymes of LDH were cleared at the same rate, *i.e.* that of LDH-I (MAHY and WACHSMUTH, 1973).

### b) Clearance of Enzymes other than LDH in LDV-Infected Mice

The plasma enzyme changes induced by LDV are quite specific and the plasma activities of several other enzymes, particularly isocitrate dehydrogenase and phosphohexose isomerase, are elevated by 8—10-fold in infected mice. On the other hand, some enzymes such as aldolase and alanine transaminase are unaffected. Studies on clearance of six enzymes other than LDH have been reported for infected and uninfected mice (see Table 13). The level of activity in the plasma of two of the enzymes (alanine transaminase and alkaline phosphatase) are not altered by LDV infection, two (aspartate transaminase and malate dehydrogenase) are increased about two-fold and two (isocitrate dehydrogenase and phosphoglucose isomerase) are grossly elevated. When the clearance of each of these enzymes

Table 13. *Clearance of Enzymes other than LDH from Plasma of LDV Infected Mice*

| Enzymes | Relative plasma activity[a] | Source of injected enzyme | Relative[b] clearance rate | Authors |
|---|---|---|---|---|
| Alanine transaminase | 1.0 | Pig heart | 1.0 | MAHY, ROWSON and PARR (1967) |
| Alkaline phosphatase | 1.0 | Calf intestine | 1.0 | NOTKINS and SCHEELE (1964) |
| Aspartate transaminase | 2.0 | Mouse erythrocytes | 0.5 | BAILEY, CLOUGH and STEARMAN (1964b) |
| Isocitrate dehydrogenase | 6.0 | Pig heart | Decreased[c] | NOTKINS and SCHEELE (1964) |
| Malate dehydrogenase | 2.0 | Mouse erythrocytes | 0.6 | BAILEY, CLOUGH and STEARMAN (1964b) |
| Phosphoglucose isomerase | 10.0 | Yeast | 0.1 | MAHY, ROWSON and PARR (1967) |

[a] Expressed relative to the activity (1.0) in normal mouse plasma.
[b] Expressed relative to the clearance rate (1.0) in normal mice.
[c] Exact value not given.

was studied, there was a close correlation between the percent reduction in clearance rate and the degree of plasma elevation (Table 13). NOTKINS and SCHEELE (1964) also studied the activities of a number of enzymes in plasma of mice following liver damage by carbon tetrachloride, which effectively increased the endogenous influx. In normal mice the activities of LDH, isocitrate dehydrogenase and malate dehydrogenase rose to very high levels after carbon tetrachloride treatment, but returned to normal quite rapidly. In LDV-infected animals the return to normal was much slower and substantial enzyme elevation persisted for several days longer. Clearly this type of experiment is hard to interpret as the result depends upon a complex interaction between the degree of liver damage (which may be a site of virus replication) and the ability of macrophages to clear the damaged cells from the circulation. But the experiment demonstrates that any disease state, infection, or chemical intoxication, that results in a release of endogenous enzymes into the circulation, may have a greater effect on LDV-infected than on normal mice.

The very large (synergistic) increases in plasma enzyme levels seen in LDV-infected tumour-bearing mice (NOTKINS and GREENFIELD, 1962a and b; RILEY, 1961, 1962a) can be adequately explained on this basis. There is considerable evidence that the amount of LDH entering the circulation is much higher in tumour-bearing than in normal mice (BURGESS and SYLVEN, 1963; JACOBSON and NISHIO, 1963; RILEY, 1963b). The increase in endogenous enzyme influx in tumour-bearing mice may cause only slight enzyme elevation if clearance is normal, but after LDV-infection the decrease in enzyme clearance would lead to accumulation of endogenous enzymes. NOTKINS (1965a) reported that enzyme clearance in tumour-bearing mice was normal, and he also presents evidence that the height of enzyme elevation in tumour-bearing mice infected with LDV was related to the degree of enzyme influx. Enzymes which increase in plasma of tumour-bearing mice, when clearance is not affected by LDV, (e.g. aldolase) do not increase synergistically in tumour-bearing animals (MAHY, ROWSON, SALAMAN, and PARR, 1964).

### c) Interaction of LDV with the Reticuloendothelial System

It is clear from the previous section that LDV infection causes an impairment of the clearance of enzymes from the circulation. This alone adequately explains the increase in plasma LDH and other enzymes which are observed in infected mice. The greater response of SJL mice to LDV infection appears to result from their greater sensitivity to blockade of enzyme clearance by the virus (CRISPENS, 1971).

One factor which has been implicated in the clearance of enzymes from the circulation is the reticuloendothelial system. Evidence was presented by WAKIM and FLEISHER (1963a and b) that blockage or stimulation of the reticuloendothelial system by zymosan or carbon inhibited or accelerated enzyme clearance in dogs.

A number of murine viruses affect reticuloendothelial system function (GLED-HILL, BILBEY, and NIVEN, 1965; MIMS, 1965), and it seemed likely LDV might also affect the reticuloendothelial system (MAHY, ROWSON, SALAMAN, and PARR, 1964).

The function of the reticuloendothelial system is normally assessed by following the rate of disappearance of carbon (usually Pelikan ink, Günther Wagner, Hannover) from the circulation after intravenous injection (HALPERN, BIOZZI, NICOL, and BILBEY, 1957; NICOL and BILBEY, 1957).

The blood carbon level can conveniently be measured optically following dilution into alkali (NICOL and BILBEY, 1957). Normal mice clear 90 per cent of the carbon from the circulation within 30 minutes, and by taking blood optical density readings at 2 to 5 minute intervals after injection the rate of clearance, and hence the phagocytic index (K) can be calculated.

The first report on reticuloendothelial system function in LDV infection was by BAILEY, STEARMAN, and CLOUGH (1963). No difference in carbon clearance was noted in LDV infected compared to normal mice, but the period for which the mice had been infected was not stated. More detailed studies (MAHY, 1964; NOTKINS and SCHEELE, 1964) showed that reticuloendothelial system function was depressed by LDV, but only during the first three days after infection (during the height of the viraemia) after which clearance of carbon returned to normal. This differs from the pattern observed for LDH clearance (Fig. 40), which does not alter until 2 days after infection and thereafter remains depressed. This result does not implicate the reticuloendothelial system in impaired enzyme clearance but it is possible that

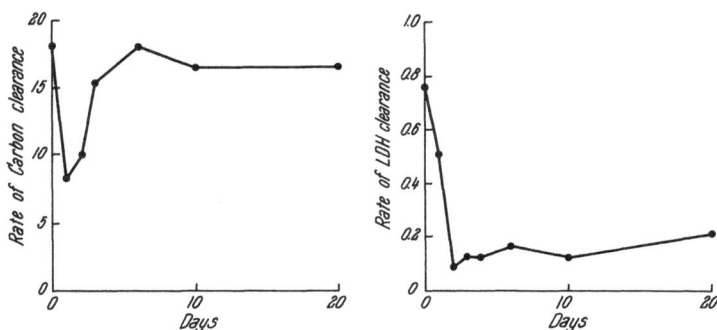

Fig. 40. Effect of LDV infection on the rate of carbon clearance (left) and LDH clearance (right) from the blood at different times after injection

carbon clearance and enzyme clearance may be handled in very different ways and even by different cells (NOTKINS, 1965a). Virus infection might still inhibit phagocytosis of enzymes by parts of the reticuloendothelial system not concerned with carbon clearance.

Table 14. *Effect of Various Treatments on Rate of Carbon Clearance in Mice*

| Treatment | Time after treatment | Effect |
|---|---|---|
| Carbon | 1—4 hours | Reduced |
| Cholesterol oleate | 1—48 hours | Reduced |
| Thorotrast | 1—48 hours | Reduced |
| Zymosan | 1—4 hours | Reduced |
| Endotoxin | 2—4 days | Stimulated |
| Stilboestrol | 1 week | Stimulated |
| Zymosan | 24—48 hours | Stimulated |

This problem was further investigated by analysing the action of various reticuloendothelial blocking and stimulating agents on plasma enzyme levels in mice (MAHY, ROWSON, PARR, and SALAMAN, 1965). The substances used, and their effects on the reticuloendothelial system are summarized in Table 14. It was found that in all cases where reticuloendothelial functions were blocked (as measured by the carbon phagocytic index), certain plasma enzyme levels increased in the plasma. These enzymes were only those affected by LDV infection. Figures 41 and 42 show the effect of LDV and cholesterol oleate, respectively, on the plasma levels of four enzymes. After LDV infection or cholesterol oleate, lactate dehydro-

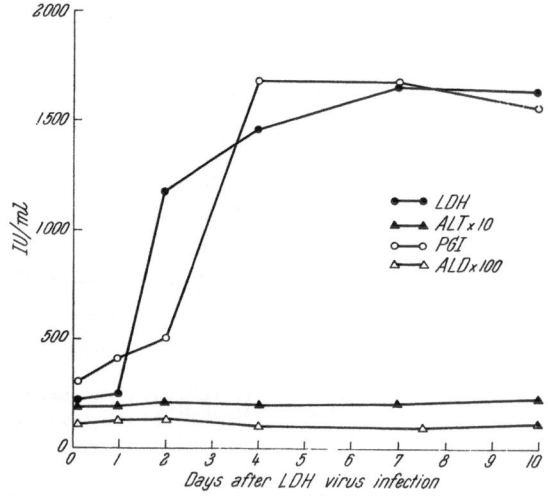

Fig. 41. Changes in plasma lactic dehydrogenase (LDH) alanine transaminase (ALT), phosphoglucose isomerase (PGI) and aldolase (ALD) levels in mice up to 10 days after infection with lactic dehydrogenase virus. Each point represents a mean value obtained from 3 to 6 mice. (From MAHY, ROWSON, PARR and SALAMAN, 1965)

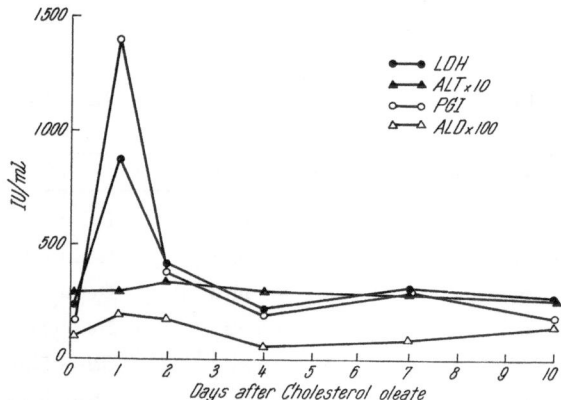

Fig. 42. Changes in plasma lactic dehydrogenase (LDH) alanine transaminase (ALT), phosphoglucose isomerase (PGI) and aldolase (ALD) levels in mice up to 10 days after an intravenous injection of 100 mg/100 g body weight cf cholesterol oleate emulsion in 1 per cent Tween 20.
Each point represents a mean value obtained from 5 mice except the values for day 0, which were obtained from 10 mice. (From MAHY, ROWSON, PARR, and SALAMAN, 1965)

genase and phosphoglucose isomerase activities increased but aldolase and alanine transaminase activities did not change. The increases in plasma enzyme levels produced by cholesterol oleate or thorotrast were temporary, in contrast to the effects of LDV. Figures 43 and 44 show the effect of thorotrast and cholesterol oleate, potent blocking agents, on plasma LDH activity in normal and LDV-infected mice.

In contrast to the effects of the blocking agents, stilboestrol, which stimulates reticuloendothelial system function (NICOL, BILBEY, CORDINGLEY, and DRUCE, 1961) reduced plasma LDH activity even in LDV-infected mice (Figs. 45 and 46)

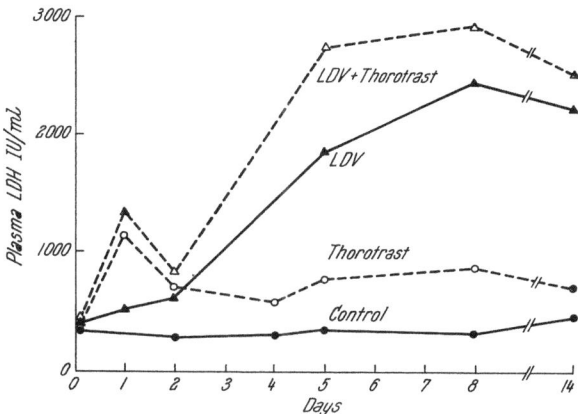

Fig. 43. Changes in plasma LDH level in groups of mice injected intraperitoneally with either 0.4 ml of normal saline on day 0 (●———●), 0.4 ml of normal saline on day 0 followed by 0.5 ml of LDV 18 hours later (▲———▲), 0.4 ml of thorotrast on day 0 (○ — — — ○) or 0.4 ml of thorotrast on day 0 followed by 0.5 ml LDV 18 hours later (△ — — — △).
Each point represents a mean value obtained from 3 to 6 mice. (From MAHY, ROWSON, PARR, and SALAMAN, 1965)

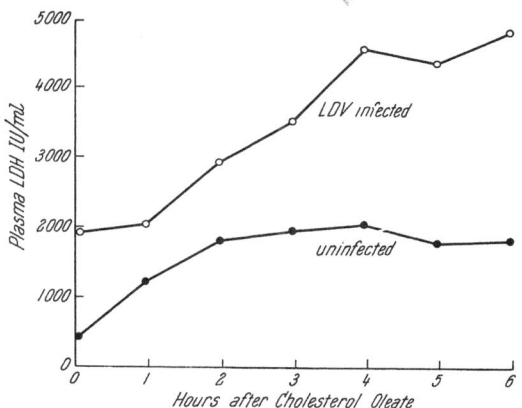

Fig. 44. Plasma LDH levels in uninfected mice and LDV infected mice (14 days previously) following an intravenous injection of cholesterol oleate, 100 mg/100 g body weight, as an emulsion in 1 per cent Tween 20. Each point represents a mean value obtained from 4 mice. (From MAHY, ROWSON, PARR, and SALAMAN, 1965)

(MAHY, ROWSON, PARR, and SALAMAN, 1965). These experiments provided considerable circumstantial evidence that the reticuloendothelial system is involved in plasma enzyme regulation, but the possibility remained that the observed effects were due to non-specific toxic action of the substances used. Later studies confirmed that alterations in enzyme clearance were responsible for the effects observed (MAHY, ROWSON, and PARR, 1967). Both cholesterol oleate

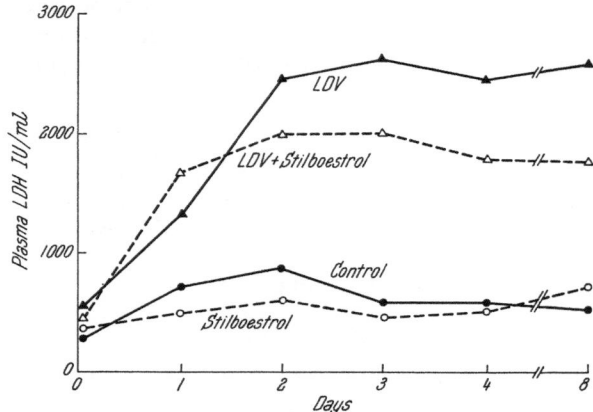

Fig. 45. Changes in plasma LDH levels in groups of mice pretreated with arachis oil (●———●), pretreated with arachis oil and injected with 1 ml LDV on day 0 (▲———▲) pretreated with stilboestrol (○ − − −○), and pretreated with stilboestrol and injected with 1 ml LDV on day 0 (△ − − − △).

Pretreatment consisted of six daily subcutaneous injections of 0.1 ml arachis oil or 0.1 stilboestrol in 0.1 ml arachis oil, commencing 1 week before virus injection. Each point represents a mean value obtained from 3 or 4 mice. (From MAHY, ROWSON, PARR, and SALAMAN, 1965)

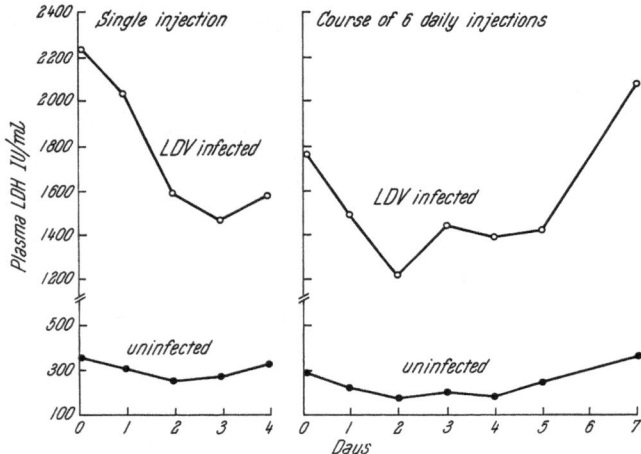

Fig. 46. Plasma LDH levels in uninfected mice and LDV (RV) infected mice (7 to 14 days previously), following a single subcutaneous injection of stilboestrol (0.1 mg in 0.1 ml arachis oil) or during a course of 6 such injections, given on days 0 to 5.

Each point represents a mean value obtained from 4 to 6 mice. (From MAHY, ROWSON, PARR, and SALAMAN, 1965)

and carbon, which impaired the function of the reticuloendothelial system assessed by carbon clearance, decreased the clearance of LDH from the circulation (Fig. 47). Stilboestrol treatment accelerated LDH clearance (Fig. 48). Oestradiol, another substance which stimulates the reticuloendothelial system, was reported to accelerate clearance of asparaginase in mice (BROOME, 1965).

These studies implicate the reticuloendothelial system in the clearance of LDH and some other enzymes from the plasma of mice. Coupled with evidence discussed elsewhere (p. 45) that the site of replication of LDV is probably in cells of the reticuloendothelial system, they support the notion that the primary pathological lesion in infected mice is an inhibition of enzyme clearance by reticuloendothelial cells.

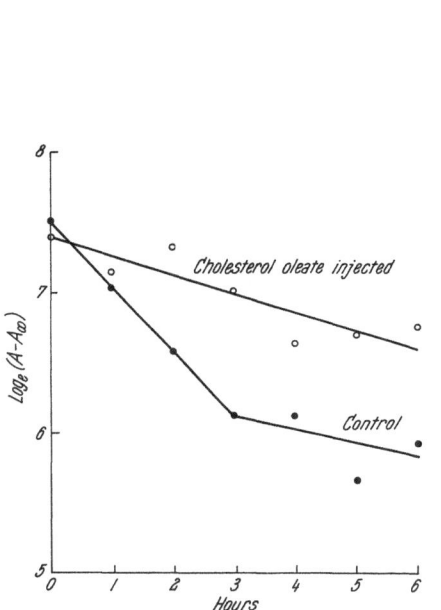

Fig. 47. Clearance of LDH from the plasma after injection of 1500 IU intravenously into normal mice (●———●) and mice injected 24 hours previously with cholesterol oleate (○———○).
Each point represents a mean value obtained from 4 mice. (From MAHY, ROWSON, and PARR, 1967)

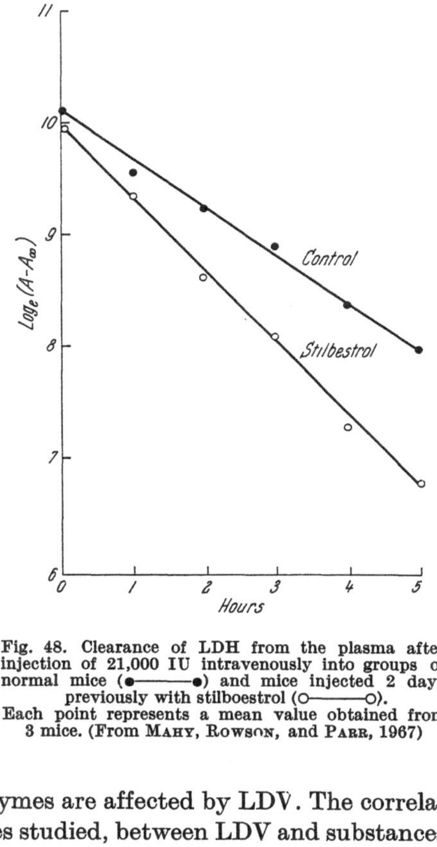

Fig. 48. Clearance of LDH from the plasma after injection of 21,000 IU intravenously into groups of normal mice (●———●) and mice injected 2 days previously with stilboestrol (○———○).
Each point represents a mean value obtained from 3 mice. (From MAHY, ROWSON, and PARR, 1967)

It is not yet clear why only certain enzymes are affected by LDV. The correlation which is found, amongst those enzymes studied, between LDV and substances causing reticuloendothelial blockade, would suggest that enzymes such as aldolase and alkaline phosphatase are handled by different cells of the reticuloendothelial system than LDV. The most informative study using LDH isoenzymes, suggests two quite different rates of clearance for LDH-I and LDH-V at high exogenous inputs (MAHY and WACHSMUTH, 1973), but below levels of $\log_e$ (A—A$_\infty$) of 6.0, LDH-V is cleared at the same rate as LDH-I. Probably two systems exist for clearance of plasma enzymes, which at least in the case of LDH appear to be charge-dependent. Cells of the fast clearance system, blocked by LDV infection, would take up only those enzymes and other particles having a particular conformation or charge. The nature of the interaction between LDV and these cells, which leads to their malfunction in infected mice, is at present unknown.

## D. Immunological Response

The prolonged viraemia in LDV infected mice suggested that neutralizing antibodies were not being formed or that they were for some reason ineffective in terminating the viraemia. Various theories were postulated to explain the apparent failure of LDV to stimulate antibody production. It was suggested (see review by NOTKINS, 1965a) that the virus was a poor antigen, perhaps because it had a lipid outer coat or an outer coat derived from the cell membrane. Another theory was that antibody formation was being prevented, possibly by multiplication of the virus in macrophages which are thought to play a role in initiating antibody production (UNANUE, 1972). LDV is known to replicate in peritoneal macrophages and it was argued that the presence of the virus in these cells could adversely affect the immunological response of the host. Alternatively, it was hypothesised that the constant outpouring of viral antigen in chronically infected animals might produce a state of immunological tolerance.

Table 15. *LDV Neutralizing Activity of Pooled Plasma from Mice 19 Weeks after Infection*

| Hours at 37° C | Residual virus infectivity ($\log_{10}$ ID$_{50}$ per ml) in plasma virus mixtures[a] | |
| --- | --- | --- |
| | Plasma[b] from | |
| | Normal mice | Infected mice |
| 0 | 4.5 | 4.5 |
| $\frac{1}{2}$ | — | 2.5 |
| 1 | 3.8 | 1.8 |
| 3 | 4.5 | 1.5 |
| 6 | 3.8 | 0.5 |
| 9 | 3.5 | 0.5 |

[a] The final plasma concentration in the mixture was 1:10. Both plasma and virus were diluted in Hanks' saline containing 20 per cent broth.
[b] Both plasma samples were heated at 58° C for 1 hour.

Eventually, however, the reason for the prolonged viraemia and the failure of simple neutralization tests to demonstrate the presence of antibodies was shown to be that a small proportion of the virus particles which combine with antibody are not neutralized but are in some way protected from neutralization on further exposure to antibody. To demonstrate LDV neutralizing antibodies it is necessary to measure the reduction in virus titre when a virus preparation is incubated with antiserum at 37° C. Using this method, neutralizing antibodies were readily demonstrated in the sera of immunized rabbits (BAILEY, CLOUGH, LOHAUS, and WRIGHT, 1965), and of chronically infected mice (ROWSON, MAHY, and BENDINELLI, 1966; NOTKINS, MAHAR, SCHEELE, and GOFFMAN, 1966; NOTKINS, 1966a and c). Before testing the sera of LDV infected mice for antibodies it is necessary to inactivate the virus which is always present in the plasma of infected mice. This can be done by heating at 58° C for one hour (Rowson, Mahy, and Bendinelli, 1966) or by exposure to ether or UV-irradiation (Notkins, Mahar, Scheele, and Goffman, 1966). Table 15 shows the results of a neutralization test in which samples of pooled plasma from normal mice and from mice injected with LDV nineteen weeks previously were mixed with virus from mice infected for 24 hours. The mixtures were incubated at 37° C and titrated for residual virus at intervals up to nine hours. The incubation caused some loss of infectivity but the difference in virus titre between the mixtures clearly shows that the plasma from the chronically infected animals had considerable neutralizing activity. However, even after nine hours incubation neutralization was not complete. That the observed neutralizing activity was not due to an interfering effect of the inactivated virus has been shown in two ways. One was to remove the virus by filtration through a Gradocol membrane of average pore diameter 62 nm and observe that the neutralizing activity was not lost (Rowson, Mahy, and Bendinelli, 1966). The other was to perform the neutralization test using a large amount of test virus which would not be neutralized to a titre below the titre of virus in the test serum. The serum from chronically infected mice contains only about $10^4$ $ID_{50}$ per ml and when such serum was added to a virus preparation containing $10^{7.7}$ $ID_{50}$ per ml and incubated at 37° C, the titre was reduced by more than 90 per cent (Notkins, Mahar, Scheele, and Goffman, 1966).

When the plasma from LDV-infected mice was tested at intervals after virus injection, neutralizing activity was first detected after 34 days and was present for at least 31 weeks (Rowson, Mahy, and Bendinelli, 1966; Notkins, Mahar, Scheele, and Goffman, 1966). Using the more sensitive technique of indirect immunofluorescence, Porter, Porter, and Deerhake (1969) were able to detect the presence of LDV antibodies as early as 6 days after infection. The serum dilution giving positive staining rose slowly from 1:10 at 6 days to 1:320 by the 28th day of infection. In a titration of the neutralizing activity in plasma from mice 48 days after infection using twofold dilutions of plasma and a constant dose of virus, the neutralizing activity did not fall until the final dilution of plasma was greater than 1:80 (Rowson, Mahy, and Bendinelli, 1966).

The fact that neutralizing activity is present in the plasma in the later stages of infection but not in the early stages is compatible with its being due to the presence of antibodies. Further support for this was that the neutralizing activity was specific for the LDH virus. No action could be demonstrated against encephalomyocarditis virus (Rowson, Mahy, and Bendinelli, 1966). The neutralizing activity was stable at —55° C for one month and on dialysis against physiological saline, but there was a considerable loss of activity on heating at 56° C for thirty minutes (Notkins, Mahar, Scheele, and Goffman, 1966). However, added mouse complement did not improve the neutralizing activity of antisera (Rowson, unpublished data). Pre-treatment of mouse antisera with goat antimouse gamma globulin caused a substantial loss of activity (Notkins, Mahar, Scheele, and Goffman, 1966).

Although in a neutralization test 99 per cent of the virus infectivity can be neutralized, a considerable amount of infectivity remains. The fact that the neutralizing activity remains constant on serum dilution up to 1:80 suggests that the cause is not a deficiency of antibody. This view is supported by an experiment in which fresh virus was added to a virus-antiserum mixture in which 99 per cent of the original virus had been neutralized. After further incubation, 99 per cent of the added virus was also neutralized, showing that an excess of antibody was present in the original mixture (NOTKINS, MAHAR, SCHEELE, and GOFFMAN, 1966).

In acutely infected mice, 99 per cent of the LDV infectivity could be neutralized, but as the infection progressed the proportion of neutralizable virus became less, and in mice forty-eight days after infection none of the circulating virus could be neutralized (ROWSON, MAHY, and BENDINELLI, 1966). This is not surprising as virus and antibody are circulating together. The presence of unneutralizable virus in the plasma of chronically infected mice and the failure to neutralize all the infectivity in the plasma of acutely infected mice with antiserum can be explained in several ways. One, and the most likely, is that of some of the virus particles become covered with a neutralization-inhibiting factor, probably an immuno-globulin. A second is that a small proportion of the virus particles is released into the plasma in some form resistant to neutralization, perhaps owing to a coating of host cell membrane. A third possibility is that the susceptible and resistant viruses are antigenically different, but, if this is so it is then necessary to explain why antibodies are not formed to both antigenic types.

That the first explanation was in fact probably the correct one was shown by NOTKINS, MAHAR, SCHEELE and GOFFMAN (1966). They found that goat anti-mouse sera or anti-mouse gamma globulin would reduce the titre of virus which had resisted neutralization by antiserum, but that goat anti-human gamma globulin was without effect. They also showed that virus sensitized to neutralization by anti-mouse serum appeared in the plasma of mice infected with LDV at about the same time as neutralizing antibody appeared. In experiments on the neutrali-zation of infective herpes simplex virus antibody complexes with anti-gamma globulin similar results have been reported (ASHE and NOTKINS, 1966; NOTKINS, 1968 and 1971b). In further experiments NOTKINS, MAGE, ASHE, and MAHAR, (1968) found that when sensitized LDV and goat anti-mouse serum were mixed at 4° C most of the viral infectivity was lost within one minute, and that further incubation at 4° or 37° C had very little effect on the residual infectivity. An excess of mouse globulin or mouse serum in the sensitized virus preparations inhibited the neutralization of the sensitized virus by the anti-mouse serum, but the presence of free mouse globulin was not the reason for the failure to obtain complete neutralization as dilution of the sensitized virus to reduce the concentra-tion of mouse serum to less than 1 per cent did not result in complete neutraliza-tion. Possible causes for the failure of anti-mouse globulin to neutralize all the infectivity in the sensitized virus preparations are: 1. the anti-viral antibody may dissociate from the virion leaving unsensitized virus which would not be suscep-tible to the action of anti-globulin, 2. the location of the antiviral antibody on the virion may be such that the anti-globulin would not cover sites critical for viral infectivity, 3. a certain percentage of the antiviral immunoglobulin used to sensitize the virus may be of a class unreactive with the particular anti-mouse globulin used, 4. heterogeneity of the anti-globulin population may result in less effective molecules blocking more effective molecules from combining with the sensitized virus, 5. some of the globulin on the virus may dissociate from it especially *in vivo* and leave infective virus. At present there is insufficient data to decide which of these possibilities is responsible for the persistence of infectivity.

The neutralization of sensitized virus depends on the specificity of the anti-immunoglobulin. Anti-IgG and anti-IgE consistently neutralized sensitized virus, anti-IgA was less effective and anti-IgM had no effect (NOTKINS, MAGE, ASHE, and MAHAR, 1968). The sensitivity of the method makes interpretation difficult. It may be that neutralization of sensitized virus by anti-IgG, IgE or IgA indicates that there are several classes of immuno-globulin on the sensitized virus, or it may be due to cross-reacting antibody in the supposedly pure antibodies.

Viraemia is a common feature in the early stages of many virus infections, but in most of them it is transitory and terminated by the appearance of neutralizing antibodies in the plasma. The occurrence of persistent viraemia in association with virus neutralizing antibodies is an unusual feature and LDV therefore presents a very interesting system for study. If on the surface of the virus there are attachment sites for antibody molecules some of which are critical and some noncritical, then attachment of antibody to the critical sites would result in neutralization of infectivity while attachment to the noncritical sites would not result in neutralization but might prevent further antibody molecules attaching to the critical sites. Anti-mouse gamma globulin could attach to the antibody molecules and this second layer of molecules could neutralize the viral infectivity. Whether or not the same antibodies are involved in neutralization and in blocking neutralization has not been determined.

Agglutination of virus particles by antiserum is one way in which the infective titre can be reduced, but NOTKINS, MAGE, ASHE, and MAHAR (1968) have shown that the infectivity of sensitized virus can be reduced by the nonprecipitating univalent Fab fragment of goat anti-mouse gamma globulin. However, the Fab fragment is less effective than the divalent gamma globulin, which could be due to the smaller size of the molecule. Further evidence against virus agglutination as the mechanism of partial neutralization is that the percentage of sensitized virus neutralized by divalent anti-mouse serum is independent of the concentration of virus.

It has been suggested that the plasma of LDV-infected mice contains infective virus particles with different physical properties. The majority of the virus particles is sedimentable on centrifugation, but there is a small fraction which is not deposited at $105,000 g$ in two hours. The virus which remains in the supernatant resists inactivation at 50° C in the presence of magnesium chloride, whereas the resuspended virus pellet contains a high proportion of virus inactivated under these conditions (CRISPENS, 1964c). Between four and six weeks after infection, the proportion of sedimentable, magnesium chloride-sensitive virus falls, and after six weeks all the infective virus is of the non-sedimentable magnesium chloride-resistant type (STARK, and CRISPENS, 1965). The close correlation between the titres of non-neutralizable and of non-sedimentable magnesium-chloride resistant virus at various stages of the infection is striking and suggests that combination with antibody may alter the properties of the virus.

## 1. Thymectomy in LDV Infection

The role of the thymus in the immune response has been extensively studied and it is known that thymectomy soon after birth impairs the ability of mice to produce antibodies. If antibody formation plays a part in controlling infection with LDV, a more severe infection would be expected in thymectomized mice, and CRISPENS (1966b) found that mice thymectomized and infected with LDV as newborn animals had, when five weeks old, a slightly higher virus titre in their serum than similarly infected but non-thymectomized mice. The virus titre was raised by less than tenfold but the LDH activity in the plasma was two to four times higher as compared with the control mice. Thymectomy when one or two weeks old had a very much reduced effect, but even in the animals thymectomized when two weeks old there was a slight potentiating effect on the raised plasma LDH level due to LDV infection. The raised LDH level in LDV infected mice is mainly due to blockade of the reticuloendothelial system (see p. 65). The more severe infection in thymectomized mice might cause a greater degree of blocking of enzyme clearance, but CRISPENS (1966b) was unable to demonstrate any difference between the rates of clearance of injected mouse LDH in intact and thymectomized LDV-infected mice. The problems involved in measuring LDH clearance at different plasma levels are discussed on page 68, but it is likely that CRISPENS' clearance tests would not detect the minor change in LDH clearance required to produce the observed effect.

LDV infection had an interesting effect on the survival of mice thymectomized at birth (CRISPENS and REY, 1967). Of eleven mice thymectomized but not infected, none survived for twenty weeks; but of forty-two thymectomized and injected with virus, five survived for twenty weeks.

## 2. Effect of LDV Infection on Immune Response to Various Antigenic Stimuli

An increased level of gamma globulin has been observed in LDV infected mice (NOTKINS, MERGENHAGEN, RIZZO, SCHEELE, and WALDMANN, 1966; NOTKINS, 1966b). In order to simplify the study of gamma globulin levels in virus-infected animals, NOTKINS and his colleagues used gnotobiotic mice. Such animals

Table 16. *Titer of γ-Globulin in Germfree Mouse Sera after Injection of LDV*

| Time after injection (days) | Titer[a] of γ-globulin in mouse sera[b] | | |
|:---:|:---:|:---:|:---:|
| | Injected with LDV | Injected with normal mouse plasma | Noninjected |
| 1 | < 16 | ND[c] | ND |
| 2 | < 16 | ND | ND |
| 3 | < 16 | ND | ND |
| 4 | < 16 | ND | ND |
| 6 | 32 | < 16 | < 16 |
| 10 | 256 | < 16 | < 16 |
| 20 | 512 | 16 | < 16 |

[a] Reciprocal of highest dilution of mouse sera giving a precipitate with goat anti-mouse γ-globulin.

[b] Pooled sera from groups of 4 to 5 mice.

[c] ND, not done.

(From NOTKINS, MERGENHAGEN, RIZZO, SCHEELE, and WALDMANN, 1969.)

have a low level of gamma globulin and on infection with LDV a slight rise was observed after six days. A more marked rise was present after ten and twenty days (see Table 16). Virus inactivated by heat, ether or ultraviolet light caused no rise in gamma globulin. If the raised gamma globulin were due to antibody it might have been expected to occur in response to the inactivated virus. This, and the fact that the clearance of certain plasma enzymes from the plasma in LDV-infected mice is impaired, suggested that the raised gamma globulin level might be due to a failure to clear it from the plasma. However, labelled mouse gamma globulin injected into normal and LDV infected mice was cleared at the same rate. It seems likely that the antigenic stimulus of the inactivated virus was insufficient and that the observed gamma globulin was in fact antibody to LDV.

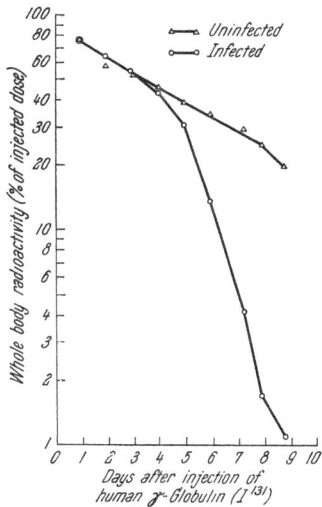

Fig. 49. Catabolism of human γ-globulin ([131]I labelled) in infected and uninfected mice. Each point represents the average of 4 mice. (From NOTKINS, MERGENHAGEN, RIZZO, SCHEELE, and WALDMANN, 1966)

When the rate of clearance of labelled human gamma globulin was followed in normal and LDV-infected mice, the rate of clearance as shown in Figure 49 was at first the same but after five days the LDV infected mice began to clear the gamma globulin at a much faster rate than the uninfected mice. The sudden increase in rate suggested that the infected animals were developing an immune response more rapidly than the normal mice. When the immune response to human gamma globulin was measured at nine days after injection, 87 per cent of LDV infected mice had responded but only 4.7 per cent of the uninfected mice. The adjuvant action of LDV was effective in mice which had been infected for sixty days but the virus had little effect given 24 hours after the gamma globulin and none when given two or six days after (NOTKINS, MERGENHAGEN, RIZZO, SCHEELE, and WALDMANN, 1966). The adjuvant action of LDV appears to be most marked when given 24 hours before the human gamma globulin, and the effect seems to be mainly an increase in IgM antibody (OLDSTONE, TISHON, and CHILLER, 1974).

Although the LDV acts as an adjuvant to antibody formation against gamma globulin, it does not affect the production of antibodies against sheep red blood cells (CRISPENS, 1968; SALAMAN and WEDDERBURN, 1966) keyhole limpet haemocyanin, or goat red blood cells (OLDSTONE, TISHON, and CHILLER, 1974).

As well as acting as an adjuvant in antibody production to injected gamma globulin, infection with LDV changed the response of mice to an injection of unaggregated gamma globulin. Adult mice injected intraperitoneally with gamma globulin which has been freed from aggregates develop immunological tolerance to the gamma globulin, instead of producing antibodies. The aggregates can be removed from a gamma globulin preparation by centrifugation at $105,000g$ for two hours or by 'biological filtration', which consists in the intravenous injection of the gamma globulin into mice and the use of their plasma containing the gamma globulin after twenty-four hours as aggregate-free material.

MERGENHAGEN, NOTKINS, and DOUGHERTY (1967) injected normal and LDV infected mice with aggregate-free human gamma globulin, and after twelve days gave them an injection of human gamma globulin in complete Freund's adjuvant. Seven days later they tested the mice for the presence of antibodies by injecting [131]I labelled human gamma globulin and measuring the rate of elimination by whole body radioactivity counting. None of the ten uninfected mice eliminated 90 per cent of the labelled protein in four days, whereas nine of the ten LDV infected mice did, indicating that they had produced antibodies. Thus LDV can prevent the development of tolerance to a soluble antigen.

The adjuvant action of LDV on antibody production to uncentrifuged gamma globulin could be demonstrated in chronically infected mice, but it was only in the acutely infected mice that the prevention of tolerance was seen. In mice injected with virus ten days previously, tolerance developed normally to an injection of unaggregated gamma globulin. The injection of virus ten days after a tolerogenic stimulus did not break the tolerance.

The way in which LDV works is not clear, but to prove that it was not due to the presence of endotoxin in the virus preparation, the virus and an endotoxin preparation were heated for thirty minutes at 80° C or exposed to UV-irradiation, and their ability to prevent tolerance developing tested. The treatment resulted in the loss of viral infectivity and ability of the virus to prevent induction of tolerance, whereas the action of the endotoxin was not inactivated.

It is interesting that LDV converts a tolerogenic stimulus into an immunogenic one only in the acute stage of infection. It is during this stage that carbon clearance is blocked, and it may be that there is a sudden disturbance of macrophage function. The virus probably replicates in these cells and soon after infection all the available cells will be infected, whereas later in the infection some balance will be established, and the rate of infection of new cells perhaps reduced.

The adjuvant action of LDV in chronically infected animals may be related to the stimulation of the formation of germinal centres which NOTKINS, MERGEN-HAGEN, RIZZO, SCHEELE, and WALDMANN (1966) described in gnotobiotic mice. In these animals the splenic white pulp consisted of densely packed, evenly distributed small lymphocytes and was essentially free of germinal centres. The red pulp contained no plasma cells. The cortical nodules of the lymph nodes were almost exclusively of the primary type, and consisted of closely packed small lymphocytes. In LDV-infected mice the spleen and lymph nodes were grossly enlarged. Histologically, the most striking alteration was the development of classical germinal centres, appearing as circular areas of pale-staining cells surrounded by a band of more darkly staining lymphocytes. Within the centres were large macrophages with cytoplasmic tingible bodies, mitotic figures, and typical 'blast' cells with large, slightly eccentric nuclei and basophilic cytoplasm. Mature plasma cells, however, were not observed. The germinal centres appeared within six days after infection but were more advanced and widespread by day 10. At 20 days the splemic white pulp had been obliterated almost completely by the development of germinal centres, and the enveloping collar of small lymphocytes had either disappeared or was very thin. Similarly, the cortical nodules of the lymph nodes contained large germinal centres and the surrounding lymphocytic band was thin and frequently incomplete.

Certain viral infections cause depression of the immune response (SALAMAN, 1969 and 1970; DENT, 1972; NOTKINS, MERGENHAGEN and HOWARD, 1970). The production of antibodies is reduced and where it has been tested the cellular immune response is also depressed. Infection with LDV enhances humoral antibody formation in mice to a soluble protein antigen but in certain cellular immune reactions, skin allograft rejection and the graft-versus-host reaction, it depresses the immune reaction (HOWARD, NOTKINS, and MERGENHAGEN, 1969). Skin allografts from $C_3H$ donors onto Balb/c hosts survived 9.6 days in the absence of LDV, while in mice injected with the virus 1 or 6 days before skin grafting, the survival time was 12.4 and 11.7 days, respectively. A similar increase in survival was observed when the virus was injected one day after grafting but given after four or six days there was no appreciable effect. The graft-versus-host reaction used by HOWARD, NOTKINS, and MERGENHAGEN (1969) consisted in injecting $F_1$ hybrid mice when eight days old with spleen cells from one of the parent strains and measuring the spleen weight of the recipients after eight days. If the recipient $F_1$ mice were infected with LDV from three to seven days before the injection of spleen cells, there was a significant reduction in the spleen weight as compared with similarly treated but uninfected control mice. The virus has little effect when given only one day before the spleen cells, and no effect if given to the donor mice one or six days before their cells were injected into uninfected $F_1$ recipients. Thus the action of the virus appears to be on the recipients rather than on the donors.

If cytophilic antibody plays an important role in allograft rejection, LDV, which replicates in macrophages, may alter their ability to react with antibody and inhibit allograft rejection. In the graft-versus-host reaction a similar process may be taking place to protect the host cells. Alternatively, the macrophages may be altered by combination with antiviral antibodies as occurs in cells infected by some other viruses (BRIER, WOHLENBERG, ROSENTHAL, MAGE, and NOTKINS, 1971).

Another experimental situation in which LDV infection reduces the immune response is in New Zealand (NZ) mice. A proportion of NZB and NZW mice develop auto-antibodies to nuclear antigen and red blood cells, and eventually develop immune-complex glomerulonephritis and autoimmune haemolytic anaemia. Infection with LDV reduces the development of antibodies and the incidence of autoimmune disease. Normally, in NZW mice the incidence of antibodies to nuclear antigen increases with age, but OLDSTONE and DIXON (1972) found that in NZW mice infected with LDV when three months old there was no subsequent increase in the proportion of mice with these antibodies. In NZB × WF₁ hybrid mice which have a higher incidence of antibodies and more severe disease, LDV infection did not make any significant difference to the incidence of antibodies but in the LDV-infected male and female (NZB × W)F₁ mice there was only a fifth to a quarter as much antibody as in the control uninfected mice. Of all the NZ mice, (NZB × W)F₁ females have the severest immune complex glomerulonephritis,

Table 17. *Effect of LDV on Contact Sensitivity to Picryl Chloride*

| Number of mice | Treatment | Sensitized with | Contact sensitivity[a] (mean ± S.D.) | P[b] |
|---|---|---|---|---|
| 6 | — | — | $2.4 \pm 1.1$ | |
| 12 | — | Picryl chloride 7 per cent | $26.1 \pm 8.0$ | |
| 12 | LDV — 1 day | Picryl chloride 7 per cent | $20.7 \pm 8.0$ | $< 0.05$ |
| 12 | LDV — 7 days | Picryl chloride 7 per cent | $21.2 \pm 6.8$ | |

[a] Expressed as increase of ear thickness 24 hours after challenge in units (1 unit = $10^{-3}$ cm).

[b] Significance of difference between the infected groups and the uninfected group.

(From ASHERSON and BENDINELLI, 1969.)

72 per cent having died by the age of nine months. Infection with LDV when four weeks old reduced the mortality to 12 per cent and even when infection was delayed to ten weeks of age the mortality at nine months was only 44 per cent (OLDSTONE and DIXON, 1972). It seems likely that LDV acts directly on the immunological system, but it is conceivable that there is a raised plasma level of DNase in the plasma of LDV-infected mice which may rapidly degrade the DNA which is stimulating the abnormal response (OLDSTONE and DIXON, 1972).

Infection with LDV appears to have little if any effect on the initiation or growth rate of most tumours (GEORGII and THORN, 1965) but it has been reported that there is an increased rate of growth of Ehrlich mouse carcinoma cells in mice infected with LDV (BAILEY, CLOUGH, and LOHAUS, 1965) and LDV has been shown to enhance the oncogenicity of mouse sarcoma virus (TURNER, EBERT, BASSIN, SPAHN, and CHIRIGOS, 1970). The development of leukaemia in Friend virus-infected mice is not affected by LDV but it does enhance spleen focus formation by Friend virus. These effects could be the result of depressed cell-mediated immunity. In contrast to these observations, RILEY (1966a) reported a decreased incidence of mammary tumours and CRISPENS (1970c) a decreased incidence of leukaemia in mice infected with LDV. The protective effect of LDV is difficult to explain but could be due to several factors.

Another aspect of cell-mediated immunity which is depressed by LDV infection is contact sensitivity. Mice can be sensitized to picryl chloride by one application of an alcoholic solution of picryl chloride to the abdominal skin, and sensitization tested for by painting the ears with picryl chloride in olive oil. The thickness of the ear is measured 24 hours after challenge. Using this procedure LDV injected 24 hours or 7 days before skin sensitization with picryl chloride depressed contact sensitivity (ASHERSON and BENDINELLI, 1969; BENDINELLI and ASHERSON, 1971) (see Table 17).

## E. Tumour Growth

LDV has been found in association with over 50 different transplantable mouse tumours (RILEY, 1968b) and it is generally thought that this is due to chance contamination, but it has been suggested by STANSLY (1965) and CRISPENS (1966c and 1970b) as an alternative explanation that the growth of tumour tissue may activate a latent LDV carried by some mice. CRISPENS induced fibrosarcomas in $C_3H/Fg$ mice by a single subcutaneous injection of 0.125 mg of methylcholanthrene in 0.2 ml of sesame oil and transplanted the tumours serially in groups of 3 or more mice. At each passage the tumours were tested for the presence of infective LDV. No virus could be demonstrated in 14 primary tumours but virus could be isolated from three tumours after the 3rd, 10th and 8th transplant generations, respectively. These results could be explained on the basis of accidental contamination, but all the animals were pretested for the virus and sterile procedures employed at all times. The possibility that LDV can be carried in a latent form deserves further study but must at present be regarded as unproved.

Infection with LDV may increase or decrease the growth rate of transplanted tumours. Soon after infection tumour growth is increased but in chronically infected mice it is decreased (MICHAELIDES and SCHLESINGER, 1974). Transplantable mouse tumours and leukaemias can be freed of LDV by passage in another species such as the rat (RILEY, 1968b) or by a period in tissue culture (BAILEY, CLOUGH, and LOHAUS, 1965). Most mouse tumours will survive in newborn rats or immunodepressed adults for 10 days by when the LDV will have disappeared. In tissue cultures the virus will die out after a similar interval (GEORGII and BRDICZKA, 1964) even if a feeder layer of mouse embryo tissue is present. The possibility that in such cell cultures the LDV has entered an eclipse phase has been suggested by RILEY (1971). In preliminary experiments he was able to obtain infective virus from a Rauscher virus-induced cell line which had lost the LDV on tissue culture passage by injecting culture fluid into mice treated with immunosuppressants. However, when more strict techniques were used to prevent accidental infection with LDV he was unable to reproduce these results (RILEY, 1974 personal communication). The immunosuppressants he used were total body X-irradiation, cortisone acetate (100 mg/kg), asparaginase (5,000 IU/kg) or anti-lymphocyte serum. Using two lines of Ehrlich mouse carcinoma cells, one freed of infective LDV by passage in tissue culture and the other contaminated with the virus, BAILEY, CLOUGH, and LOHAUS (1965) noticed that the tumour cells free of virus did not cause such rapid abdominal distension on intraperitoneal injection as the virus contaminated cells. The accelerated growth rate was observed when LDV contaminated cells were injected into normal mice and when virus-free cells were injected into mice infected with the virus 4 days previously. Unfortunately in view of the extremely high rate of replication of LDV it is not possible to conclude from this observation whether its action is on the tumour cells or the host.

RILEY (1963 b) observed a similar acceleration of tumour growth when he added LDV to a virus-free methyl cholanthrene-induced tumour but in subsequent studies he found that the tumour growth rate sometimes appeared to be inhibited by the added virus and he came to the conclusion that LDV did not have a reproducible or predictable influence on the growth rate (RILEY, 1968 b). PLAGEMANN and SWIM (1963 and 1966 b) were also unable to demonstrate any difference in growth rate when virus-free tumours were grown in normal or LDV infected mice. They used sarcoma 180 and hepatomas 129 and 134, which they had freed of virus by passage *in vitro*.

The reason for the somewhat conflicting reports on the effect of infection with LDV on the growth of transplantable tumours may be that the virus has a weak effect seen only when a small number of cells are injected and that the action of the virus is to increase tumour growth soon after infection but to decrease it in chronically infected mice. MICHAELIDES and SCHLESINGER (1974) injected different doses of the plasmacytoma MOPC-315 subcutaneously into uninfected mice and mice infected 24 hours previously with LDV. When they injected $4 \times 10^5$ tumour cells, tumours appeared more rapidly and more mice developed tumours in the LDV-infected than in the control group (100 per cent at 22 days compared with 25 per cent at 36 days for the control group). When they used mice infected with LDV 3 weeks previously, tumours appeared later and in fewer mice than in the control group. Mice infected for 5 months with LDV showed no difference from the control mice in their susceptibility to tumour cell growth.

A number of both oncogenic and non-oncogenic viruses have been shown to influence the development of tumours induced by other viruses and non-viral carcinogens (ROE and ROWSON, 1968). LDV has an action on the reticuloendothelial system which has a role in the development of tumours (OLD, BENACERRAF, CLARKE, CARSWELL, and STOCKERT, 1961) and so it could well be expected to have an effect on tumour incidence and growth. However, LDV has not been found to have any influence on the development of spontaneous tumours with the exception of "spontaneous" mammary tumours and possibly leukaemia. RILEY (1966 a) compared the incidence of mammary carcinoma developing in two groups of non-parous $C_3H/HeJ$ mice, one free of LDV and the other injected with the virus when 56 days old. The mice were observed for about 18 months, and in that time there was a 90 per cent incidence of mammary tumours in the controls, in contrast to a 53 per cent incidence in the virus injected mice. The time required for 50 per cent of the LDV-infected animals to produce tumours was 484 days as compared with 353 days for the control group. There was no observable difference in body weight between the control and infected mice during the period before tumour development. Similar results were obtained using $C_3H \times I$ females, although the protective effect of LDV was less striking in these nonparous $F_1$ mice, but this may have been because the virus was not injected until the mice were from 150 to 177 days old (RILEY, 1968 b). Intensive breeding of $C_3HeJ$ mice lessened the ultimate protective effect of LDV observed in the nonparous animals, the final tumour incidence being 100 per cent in both infected and control animals. However, even with intensive breeding there was a significant difference in the time at which tumours appeared. When the mice were 294 days old, the tumour incidence was 83 per cent in LDV-free mice, compared with 36 per cent in the infected mice. The median latent period to tumour development was 310 days in the infected animals and 267 days in the controls. CRISPENS (1970c) followed 120 C₃H/Fg mice injected with LDV as newborns and 71 control mice similarly injected with Eagle's basal medium. The leukaemia incidence was 49 per cent in the controls and 38 per cent in the infected mice. The difference was mainly due to a marked decrease in the incidence of leukaemia among the LDV-injected males (controls 75 per cent, LDV-infected 42 per cent). The mean latent period for the control mice was 367 days and for the virus infected mice 442 days. Infection with LDV is reported to reduce the severity of the leukocytic response to Friend virus infection (RILEY, LOVELESS, FITZMAURICE, SMULLYAN, and FISCHER, 1967). The importance of using LDV-free stock in experiments on mammary tumour and leukaemia development is obvious, and a failure to appreciate this in the past may account for some of the discrepancies reported in the literature.

LDV has been shown to have no effect on the development of leukaemia in mice injected with Moloney leukaemia virus when 3 to 4 days old (ROWSON, ADAMS, and SALAMAN, 1963). The incidence and latent period were unaffected, no matter whether the virus was given two days before, at the same time, or two days after the leukaemia virus. LDV is also reported not to influence the development of leukaemia following X-irradiation (RILEY, 1968b). Although LDV does not affect the development of leukaemia, it does enhance spleen focus formation by Friend virus if injected intravenously 2 days before the Friend virus. Injected 5 days before or at the same time as the Friend virus it causes no enhancement (STEEVES, MIRAND, THOMSON, and AVILA, 1969). RILEY and FITZMAURICE (1973) found that on passage *in vitro* a line of (Rauscher leukaemia virus produced) cells, which had previously been highly leukaemogenic, became free of LDV and lost the ability to produce typical Rauscher leukaemia readily although they continued to produce Rauscher virus. When mice inoculated with this poorly leukaemogenic material were injected with LDV they rapidly developed leukaemia. It seems that under certain conditions LDV can increase the leukaemogenic potential of certain viruses but it is likely that its action is to depress cell-mediated immunity rather than to aid cell transformation.

LDV has also been shown to enhance the oncogenicity of both the Harvey and Moloney strains of murine sarcoma virus (MSV) (TURNER, EBERT, BASSIN, SPAHN, and CHIRIGOS, 1970). Adult mice inoculated with LDV 3 days before inoculation with MSV showed substantially increased tumour incidence, reduced frequency of tumour regression and reduced median survival time as compared to control animals give MSV alone. When the two viruses were injected at the same time, LDV showed no enhancement of MSV infection. Tumour extracts from mice inoculated with MSV alone showed no focus-forming and tumour-inducing activity whereas extracts of tumours from dually infected mice contained focus-forming and tumour-inducing activity. The mechanism by which LDV potentiates the activity of MSV is not clear but may be related to the depression of cell-mediated immunity by LDV (HOWARD, NOTKINS, and MERGENHAGEN, 1969). There is no evidence for a change in the genome of the MSV extracted from the tumours of the dually infected mice; the virus behaves in the same way as the stock MSV being more potent in mice previously infected with LDV than in LDV-free animals.

The development of primary tumours following the injection of 1 mg of 20 methylcholanthrene into DBA/2 mice was unaffected by an injection of LDV given at the same time (RILEY, 1968b).

LDV appears to have little if any effect on the initiation or development of most tumours, but it has a very marked potentiating effect on the plasma enzyme changes produced by tumours (GEORGII, THORN, and WRBA, 1966b; ADAMS, ROWSON, and SALAMAN, 1961; MAHY, ROWSON, SALAMAN, and PARR, 1964; NOTKINS, 1965a; EBERT, CHIRIGOS, FIELDS, and ELLSWORTH, 1967). This synergistic effect almost certainly results from blocking of the normal plasma enzyme clearing system (see p. 65), and not from any direct action of the virus on the tumour cells. The very high plasma enzyme levels in LDV-infected tumour-bearing mice do not, in most cases, adversely affect tumour growth. However, some tumour cells, unable to synthesize asparagine and dependent on an exterior source of this amino acid, are inhibited by the injection of L. asparaginase. In mice, the clearance of injected L. asparaginase from the plasma is reduced by infection with LDV and the therapeutic effect of the enzyme is considerably improved (RILEY, CAMPBELL, and STOCK, 1970; RILEY, 1969 and 1970; RILEY, SPECKMAN, FITZMAURICE, and LULHAM, 1970; SPECKMAN, RILEY, and TESCHNER, 1970; RILEY, SPECKMAN, FITZMAURICE, ROBERTS, HOLCENBERG, and DOLOWY, 1974). Using EARAD-I leukaemia cells freed of LDV by passage in tissue culture as the test tumour, an injection of 100 I.U. of EC-2 L. asparaginase on the seventh or ninth day after tumour inoculation had no effect on the incidence or time of death from leukaemia. However, if LDV was injected on the fourth day after tumour inoculation, a similar dose of asparaginase reduced the number of deaths by day 40 from 100 per cent to 5 per cent (RILEY, 1968a). Attention was drawn to the role of LDV in asparaginase therapy by the paradoxical finding that the enzyme was more effective when administered against tumour cells implanted 7 days previously than when given 1 hour after the tumour cells (OLD, IRITANI, STOCKERT, BOYSE, and CAMPBELL, 1968). In the latter case, most of the enzyme would be eliminated from the plasma prior to blocking of enzyme clearance by the LDH virus, which was present in most of the mouse tumours used in experiments, showing the therapeutic value of asparaginase (RILEY, CAMPBELL, and STOCK, 1970). That tumours reduced the clearance of asparaginase was noted by BROOME (1968) who presumably did not appreciate that it was due to the LDH virus [see also BOYD and PHILLIPS (1971) and PHILLIPS and BOYD (1969)]. The changes in plasma amino acid levels following an injection of asparaginase are not confined to asparagine and glutamine but in the LDV-free mouse the changes are very small. However, in LDV-infected animals the secondary effects of asparaginase are potentiated and may be of importance in suppressing tumour growth (RILEY, SPECKMAN, and FITZMAURICE 1970a and b and 1971; SPECKMAN and RILEY, 1971; RILEY, SPECKMAN, FITZMAURICE, ROBERTS, HOLCENBERG, and DOLOWAY, 1972 and SPECKMAN and RILEY, 1972).

The clearance of LDH isoenzymes is dependent on charge (see p. 70), and it is interesting to speculate that an alteration in the charge on the asparaginase molecule might also lead to a decrease in clearance rate from the plasma. If this could be accomplished, the potential value of asparaginase therapy for an aspara-gine-dependent tumour might be greatly enhanced.

## F. Histological Changes

The only macroscopic changes demonstrable in mice after infection with LDV are an increase in spleen weight, lymphoid hyperplasia and a slight transitory fall in thymus weight (SANTISTEBAN, RILEY, and FITZMAURICE, 1972; RILEY, HUERTO,

Table 18. *Spleen Weight in Groups of 5 BALB/c Mice at Different Times after Infection with LDV*

| Time after injection of LDV (days) | Spleen weight mg ± standard deviation | |
| --- | --- | --- |
| | Uninfected mice | Infected with LDV |
| 7 | 90±17 | 156±20 |
| 14 | 118±8 | 141±11 |
| 21 | 106±7 | 167±59 |

LILLY, BARDELL, LOVELESS, and FITZMAURICE, 1961; RILEY, 1964; PROFFITT and CONGDON, 1970; PROFFITT, CONGDON, and TYNDALL, 1972; SNODGRASS, LOWREY, and HANNA, 1972). Table 18 shows the mean spleen weight in groups of 5 BALB/c female mice at weekly intervals after the intravenous injection of LDV. The degree of splenomegaly produced by the virus is slight but significant when compared with the control animals. Of the 15 infected mice in Table 18 only one had a spleen weighing over 200 mg. POPE and ROWE (1964) examined 20 mice one month after virus inoculation and found 5 with spleens weighing over 200 mg. NOTKINS (1965a) found only 21 of 55 infected mice with spleens weighing 30 per cent more than normal. He observed that the splenomegaly occurred within 72 hours of infection and persisted for at least a month. It was the increase in spleen size which led POPE (1963) to recognize the presence of the WMI strain of LDV in the mice he had injected with material from wild mice. He did not weigh the spleens of his mice but assessed their size by the product of their length and breadth. It is thus difficult to compare his results with spleen weights given by other workers.

The fall in thymus weight commences within 24 hours of injection of LDV and is linear with time for the first 96 hours (SANTISTEBAN, RILEY, and FITZMAURICE, 1972). The maximum effect is seen on day 3 or 4 when the thymus has lost 30 to 40 per cent of its mass. By day 8 the thymus weight has returned to a level above that of the controls (PROFFITT and CONGDON, 1970).

The increase in spleen weight is evident within 24 hours of infection but the increase in lymph node mass is more gradual and not clearly significant until the third day. Few typical germinal centres are seen until day 16 after infection.

The histological changes in LDV-infected mice are not dramatic in spite of the rapid virus replication taking place, and for some years routine histological examination of the tissues from LDV-infected mice failed to reveal any change associated with the infection in lungs, spleen, thymus, brain, heart, kidneys or liver (BAILEY, CLOUGH, and STEARMAN, 1964a; GEORGII, KROTH, and BAYERLE, 1962). However, there is splenomegaly and lymph node enlargement in LDV infected mice, and more detailed study of the lymphoid tissue has revealed certain interesting changes. There is hyperplasia of the germinal centres and a reduction in the numbers of lymphocytes in the thymus-dependent areas (PROFFITT, CONGDON, and TYNDALL, 1972; SNODGRASS, LOWREY, and HANNA, 1972). There is congestion with erythrocytes and numerous erythropoietic foci in the red pulp of the spleen and this appears to be the major factor causing the early increase in spleen weight (SNODGRASS, LOWREY, and HANNA, 1972).

The germinal centre hyperplasia is most marked in gnotobiotic mice because of their lack of germinal centres before infection (NOTKINS, MERGENHAGEN, RIZZO, SCHEELE, and WALDMANN, 1966). The germinal centres are cellular compartments in the lymphatic tissue and the functions attributed to them include antigen trapping, immunocyte proliferation and antibody production (CONGDON, 1969). C-type leukaemia virus particles tend to concentrate along the surfaces of the membrane infoldings of dendritic reticular cells (antigen-retaining cells) in the germinal centres. LDV also appears to accumulate on the membrane infoldings in the same way (Fig. 16). Six hours after the injection of LDV, SNODGRASS and HANNA (1970) found many virus particles in close intercellular association with phagocytic reticular cells in the marginal zone. Intercellular virus particles were frequently aligned along the plasmalemma of their cells, as if associated with receptor sites. Only a few particles were seen within single membrane-bound intracellular vesicles and only complete virus particles were seen. Small extravesicular particles were not detected in the cytoplasm of these macrophages. The number of virus particles in the marginal zone decreased after 24 hours and by 4 days from the time of infection only a few particles could be found.

The thymic-dependent areas of lymphatic tissue are those areas which are depleted of lymphocytes in mice thymectomized at birth. In these areas following injection of LDV there was necrosis of cells observable after 24 hours but most marked after 48 hours. The reticulum became prominent and many macrophages containing debris were present. Four days after infection the nuclear debris had been cleared and only a few macrophages were present, there was no remaining evidence of cell death or of repopulation to the preinfection status. Virus particles did not appear in the thymic-dependent area surrounding the central artery as early as in the marginal zone. They were most numerous 2 days after infection and were localized intercellularly, associated with phagocytic cells which were morphologically the same as those in the marginal zone (HANNA, SZAKAL, and TYNDALL, 1970; HANNA, WALBURG, TYNDALL, and SNODGRASS, 1970; PROFFITT, CONGDON, and TYNDALL, 1972).

The role of the adrenals in the pathology of LDV infection has been investigated by SANTISTEBAN and his colleagues (SANTISTEBAN, RILEY, and FITZMAURICE, 1972; SANTISTEBAN, RILEY, and WILLHIGHT, 1970; SPECKMAN, RILEY, SANTISTEBAN, KIRK, and BREDBERG, 1974). They found that adrenalectomy before infection with LDV prevents the involution of the thymus observed in intact controls, whereas the increase in spleen and lymph node weight is greater (Figs. 50 and 51). The more marked splenomegaly in the infected adrenalectomized mice is compatible with the two types of change taking place — atrophy of the thymic-dependent areas prevented by adrenalectomy and hypertrophy of the germinal centres which is not affected. SANTISTEBAN, RILEY, and FITZMAURICE (1972) hypothesize that the virus increases the level of the circulating adrenal cortical hormones which causes the thymic involution and necrosis in the thymic-

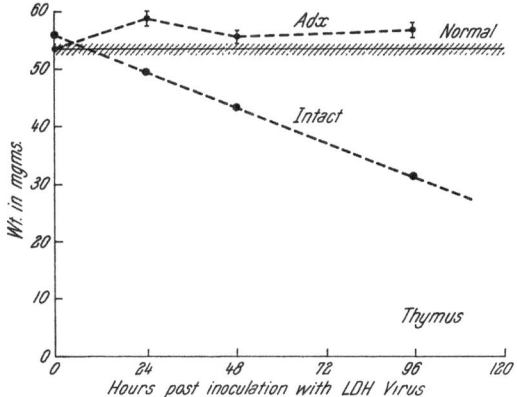

Fig. 50. Thymus weight of intact and adrenalectomized mice at 24, 48 and 96 hours following injection of LDV. (From SANTISTEBAN, RILEY, and FITZMAURICE, 1972)

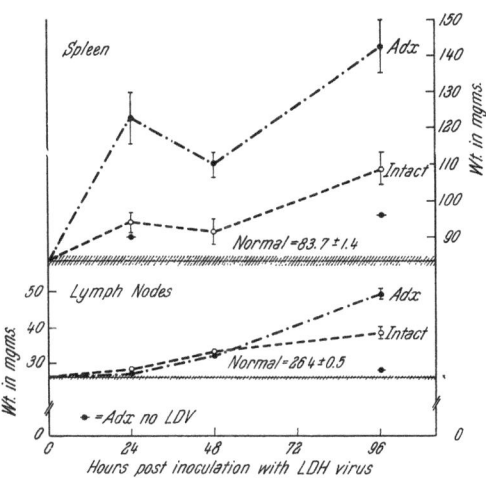

Fig. 51. Spleen and lymph node weights of intact and adrenalectomized mice at 24, 48 and 96 hours following injection of LDV. (From SANTISTEBAN, RILEY, and FITZMAURICE, 1972)

dependent areas of the spleen. Subjection of animals to stress is known to cause involution of the thymus and this can be prevented by adrenalectomy. That the effect of the LDV injection was not simply due to the manipulation, is clear from the finding that sham-injected intact animals showed no thymic involution. How the virus acts to increase the adrenal function has not been investigated, but virus replication as judged by the level of viraemia is not affected by adrenalectomy

(SANTISTEBAN, RILEY, and FITZMAURICE, 1972). SNODGRASS, LOWREY, and HANNA (1972), in contrast to SANTISTEBAN and his colleagues, did not find that adrenalectomy prevented the fall in thymic weight following infection with LDV (Fig. 52). In their experiments there was no significant difference in the way LDV affected mice when the source of adrenal hormones was removed. They hypothesize that the fall in thymic weight may be due to intrathymic lymphocytes leaving to replace the loss of thymus-dependent lymphocytes from the blood and thymus-dependent areas of the spleen and lymph nodes. The destruction of thymus-dependent lymphocytes may be directly caused by the virus or by a soluble virus

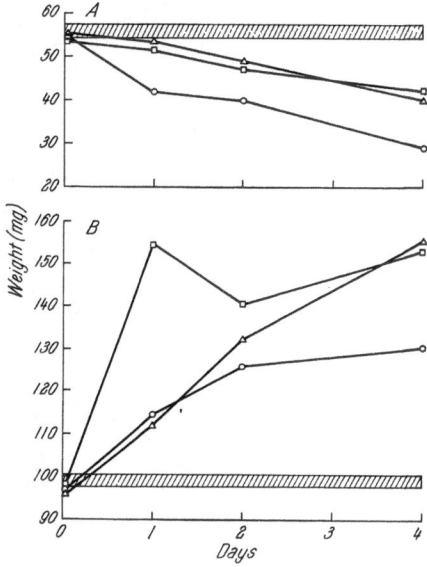

Fig. 52. (A) Thymus and (B) spleen weight changes in normal (△), adrenalectomized (□) and shamoperated (○) mice after inoculation with LDV. (From SNODGRASS, LOWREY, and HANNA, 1972)

product which does not cross the thymus-blood barrier. If LDV is injected directly into the thymus, there is destruction of the lymphocytes in the cortex. This response is similar to that occurring in other lymphoid organs when the virus is injected by the usual routes (SNODGRASS, LOWREY, and HANNA, 1972). Another possible mechanism for the destruction of thymus-dependent lymphocytes, postulated by SNODGRASS, LOWREY, and HANNA (1972), is that a cell-mediated immune reaction is mounted against the antigenically altered membranes of the phagocytic cells of the reticulum in which the virus probably replicates. This cell-mediated response could destroy the thymus-dependent lymphocytes and the cells in which the virus replicates. However, the speed of the response after infection seems too rapid, and when the thymus-dependent areas are repopulated they are not destroyed.

Glomerulonephritis associated with the deposition of virus-antibody-complement complexes in the glomeruli has been described in mice chronically infected with lymphocytic choriomeningitis virus (OLDSTONE and DIXON, 1969) and mouse sarcoma virus (HIRSCH, ALLISON, and HARVEY, 1969). These viruses resemble

LDV in giving rise to a chronic infection in which infective virus-antibody complexes are present in the plasma for months. The trapping of the circulating complexes in the glomeruli is thought to be the cause of the nephritis. In LDV-infected mice significant deposits of IgG and complement can be demonstrated in a granular-to-lumpy distribution along the glomerular capillary walls seven days

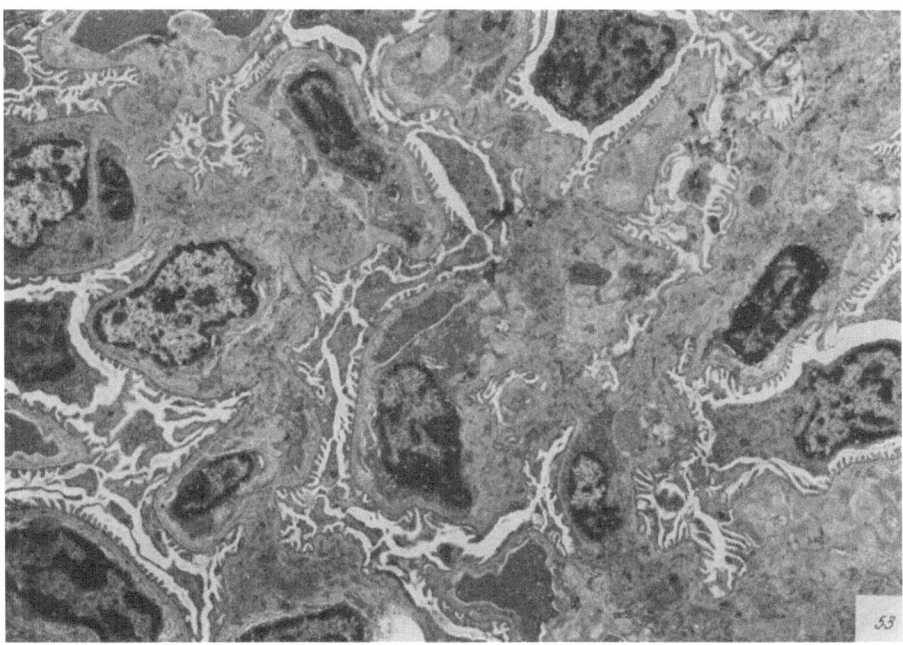

Fig. 53. Section of kidney 24 hours after injection of LDV.
Almost all the cells seen are endothelial cells which are markedly swollen to fill the lumen of the glomerular capillaries. A dark exudate is present between many endothelial cells and basement membranes, which are normal.
Magnification × 4,000

after infection (PORTER and PORTER, 1971). With time, the deposits become more marked, but there is an increase in the number of control mice not infected with LDV showing antibody deposits in the glomeruli (OLDSTONE and DIXON, 1971). The deposits in the control mice are presumably due to chance infections or endogenous murine leukaemia virus. After 7.5 or 8 months from the time of infection with LDV, the histopathological changes in the glomeruli were minimal and limited to an increase in mesangial cells with a corresponding slight increase in the thickening of the glomerular capillary wall. Electron microscopic studies of the renal tissue of mice infected with LDV (ROWSON, MICHAELS, and HURST, 1974) have shown swelling of the capillary endothelial cells of the glomeruli as early as 24 hours after infection (Fig. 53). These changes persisted for at least 3 months but did not progress in severity. It is surprising that the persistent presence of virus-antibody-complement complexes in the glomeruli, and definite histological changes, do not lead to the severe type of nephritis seen in other chronic virus infections. The reason for this must remain in doubt until more is known of the reasons for the damage caused by the deposits. OLDSTONE and DIXON (1971) found that some strains of mice were more likely than others to develop deposits in their glomeruli. Six weeks after LDV infection the incidence of deposits in the glomeruli was 87 per cent in C3H, 40 per cent in SWR/J and 20 per cent in SW mice.

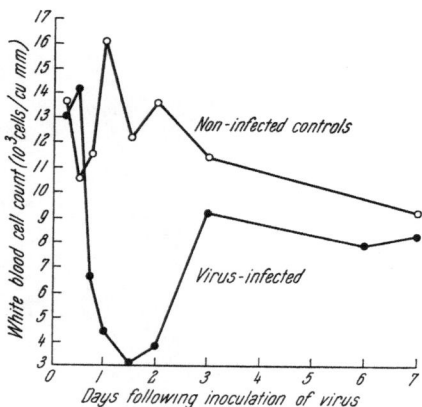

Fig. 54. Leukopenia following injection of LDV

RILEY (1968b) has observed a substantial but transitory fall in the total white blood cell count 24 hours after injection of LDV (Fig. 54). The leukopenia lasted for only about 24 hours, and by the third day after infection the white cell count was the same in the infected and control animals. BAILEY, STEARMAN, and CLOUGH

Table 19. *Haematocrits and White Blood Cell Counts in Normal and Infected Mice*

| Type of mouse | Number of mice | Mean haematocrit (%)[a] | Number of mice | Mean WBC/mm[3a] |
|---|---|---|---|---|
| Normal | 90 | 50.17±.52 | 16 | 8543±773 |
| Infected | 80 | 47.14±.47 p≪.001 | 13 | 9430±1139 p>.1 |

[a] ± Standard error of mean.

(From BAILEY, STEARMAN, and CLOUGH, 1963.)

(1963) did not observe any difference in the white blood cell count between normal and LDV infected mice, but they did not examine blood 24 and 48 hours after infection. They did, however, record a small but significant depression of the packed red blood cell volume (see Table 19). The slight fall in haematocrit has been observed 3 and 7 days after infection (RILEY, 1968b) but the cause has not been investigated. In mice with anaemia due to repeated blood sampling no difference was observed in the rate at which normal and LDV-infected mice recovered (BAILEY, CLOUGH and STEARMAN, 1964a). Infection with LDV has been shown to increase the rate at which injected $^{59}$Fe is incorporated into the peripheral erythrocytes (SNODGRASS, YUHAS, and HANNA, 1973).

# VII. Ecology

Infection with LDV occurs spontaneously in both wild and laboratory mice. All strains of mice are susceptible but no other species has been found naturally infected or infectable (see p. 52).

LDV has been isolated from wild mice in Australia (POPE, 1961), U.S.A. (POPE and ROWE, 1964), Germany (GEORGII and KIRSCHENHOFER, 1965) and England (ROWSON, 1963; FIELD and ADAMS, 1968). No systematic study of the infection in wild mice has been reported and it is not possible to say, with any certainty, how common the infection is. However, most reported isolations from wild mice were made on small numbers of animals and a high proportion were infected. In Maryland, U.S.A., 8 mice were examined and 4 were infected. In Germany 40 mice were studied; nine had raised LDH levels but 7 of these were due to non-specific causes. From the other 2 mice a virus was isolated which had all the characteristics of LDV. In England, 19 mice trapped in Hampshire were tested and 12 were infected, while of 21 caught in Northumberland, 9 were infected. This suggests that infection with LDV is common among wild mice, but it is not to be found in all wild colonies. We found no infected mice in a sample of 15 mice trapped in the London Docks, and PLAGEMANN, GREGORY, SWIM, and CHAN (1963) did not isolate the virus from several wild mice they examined.

Laboratory mouse colonies appear much less likely to be infected with LDV than wild mice, but there are three reports of infection among mice not known to have been exposed to infected animals. PLAGEMANN, GREGORY, SWIM, and CHAN (1963) found all of the 30 mice they tested from one Canadian laboratory were infected. RILEY (1963b) found a number of infected mice in batches of animals received from various breeders. He also found infected mice in "germ-free" stock (RILEY, 1965).

Mice infected with LDV excrete the virus in their faeces, urine and milk (PLAGEMANN, GREGORY, SWIM, and CHAN, 1963; NOTKINS, 1965a; CRISPENS, 1964b and d). The virus is also present in the mouth and is probably secreted in the saliva (CRISPENS, 1964b; NOTKINS, 1965a). NOTKINS (1965a) titrated the infectivity in urine, faeces, saliva and milk at various times after infection. The highest virus titres were obtained 24 hours after infection, in the milk and faeces. The titre in the milk was $10^{7.2}$ $ID_{50}$/ml and that in the faeces $10^{5.9}$ $ID_{50}$/ml. The faeces continued to be infective for at least 135 days but virus was not detected in the urine for more than 16 days. The milk was infected when examined for the last time 16 days after infection. CRISPENS (1964b) found virus in the saliva, urine and faeces 36 hours after infection but at 5 weeks it was only present in the faeces. In the milk, CRISPENS (1965b) found infective virus present for at least 63 days, but the titre fell from $10^{5.8}$ $ID_{50}$/ml, twenty four hours after infection, to $10^{4.3}$ $ID_{50}$/ml at 63 days.

Mice are readily infected with LDV if it is injected intravenously, intraperitoneally, intramuscularly, intracerebrally or subcutaneously. Dermal application of the virus has been reported to cause infection (RILEY, LILLY, HUERTO, and BARDELL, 1960; RILEY, 1963b) but it is probably necessary for infection by this route to have minor skin abrasions (NOTKINS, 1965a). Infection follows oral administration provided a large dose is given. NOTKINS and SCHEELE (1963) took groups of

10 mice and deprived them of water for 24 hours. He then gave them 20 to 50 ml of distilled water containing virus which they drank in 6 to 12 hours. When the virus titre in the drinking water was $10^{6.4}$ $ID_{50}$/ml, no mice were infected but when the titre was increased to $10^{8.8}$ $ID_{50}$/ml, approximately half the mice exposed were infected. In another experiment they used a plastic tube to deliver the virus-containing water directly into the oral pharynx. Given in this way, 0.2 ml of water containing $10^{8.8}$ $ID_{50}$/ml infected 10 out of 10 mice used.

Cross-infection between infected and uninfected mice in the same cage has been observed (RILEY, HUERTO, LILLY, and BARDELL, 1961; HILL, TANAKA, and ROBERTS, 1962; PLAGEMANN, GREGORY, SWIM, and CHAN, 1963; CRISPENS, 1964b and d) but transmission of the infection is somewhat irregular. In one experiment, 4 out of 5 mice put into a cage with infected mice were infected after 32 days while in another experiment 20 uninfected mice in a cage with 5 infected mice were uninfected after a similar interval. These mice were subsequently shown not to be immune to infection (PLAGEMANN, GREGORY, SWIM, and CHAN, 1963). Similar but rather more regular transmission was obtained by CRISPENS (1964b). He took groups of 5 mice and injected virus into one, two, three or four of them, and tested the uninjected mice for signs of infection after one, three, five and seven weeks. In the cages where three or four mice were injected, the uninjected mice were infected after one week but in the cages where only one or two mice were injected, none of the uninjected mice were infected after one week and it was not until five weeks that they were all infected. These results suggest the rate of transmission is related to the ratio of infected to uninfected animals in a cage.

Faeces appear to be the main source of virus for the spread of the infection under natural conditions, but as mice are not readily infected with small doses of virus by mouth, biting during the early days of the infection, when virus is present in the saliva, may be an important method of transmission. However, CRISPENS (1964b) found no evidence for this. NOTKINS, SCHEELE, and SCHERP (1964) found that the infection spread much more rapidly in general purpose Swiss mice, where there was much more fighting than in other strains where fighting was much less frequent. Also, transmission was more frequent between the older male Swiss mice than between females and young males, where signs of biting were less evident. To prevent biting, the Swiss mice were made partially edentulous by extraction of the upper incisors and amputation of the lower incisors at the gum line. This procedure reduced the cross infection rate from 100 per cent to less than 5 per cent and showed the importance of biting in the transmission of LDV but it did not answer the question as to whether the virus was being transmitted to the normal animals by inoculation of infected saliva or whether the normal animals were being infected as a result of biting and ingesting virus infected tissue. To answer this question, uninfected mice without incisors were exposed to infected mice with incisors and the transmission rate determined. The mice without incisors became infected, supporting the idea that virus is transmitted by inoculation of infected saliva. However, when normal mice with incisors were exposed to infected mice without incisors, 75 per cent of the normal animals became infected, suggesting that infection may also result from ingestion of infected tissue. The high virus titre in the blood soon after infection would provide a sufficient concentration of virus to produce infection by the oral route. Further evidence that cannibalism may be a factor in the transmission of LDV is that when a dead infected mouse is placed in a cage with uninfected mice, the latter only become infected if the dead mouse is eaten (NOTKINS, SCHEELE, and SCHERP, 1964).

Transmission between mice in adjacent cages has been reported but is infrequent (PLAGEMANN, GREGORY, SWIM, and CHAN, 1963; NOTKINS, 1963a) and if the mice are separated by a one-inch air space and transmission of excreta between the cages is prevented, cross-infection does not take place (CRISPENS, 1964b).

Transmission of LDV from infected parents to their young occurred with a frequency of over 90 per cent if the females were infected with virus during pregnancy and with a frequency of 50 per cent if the virus was injected into the lactating mouse within 48 hours of parturition (NOTKINS and SCHEELE, 1963b; CRISPENS, 1964a and 1965b). When both parents were infected 7 days before mating the transmission rate to the young varied between less than one per cent (NOTKINS and SCHEELE, 1963b; CRISPENS, 1964b) 44 per cent (CRISPENS, 1965b) and 59 per cent (CRISPENS, 1967a). In these experiments the young were examined when 3 to 5 weeks old and infection could have occurred at any time but as mice are not readily infected from their cage-mates in the absence of fighting it seems likely that the young of mothers infected during lactation were infected via the milk. The very high incidence of infection in the young of mothers infected during pregnancy, as compared with those whose mothers were infected after parturition, suggests that the virus crosses the placenta during the acute phase of the infection when the plasma virus titre is high. In support of this theory, CRISPENS (1965b) found that newborn mice which were separated from their infected mothers immediately after birth were infected, and GEORGII, LENZ, and ZOBEL (1964) found that the embryos were infected 72 hours after the mother was injected with virus. The difficulty of obtaining embryos free of contamination by the mother's body fluids is obvious but that GEORGII and his colleagues were successful in doing this is suggested by the fact that embryos removed 24 hours after the mother was infected, were not infected, although at this time the maternal plasma virus titre would be very high. In this work, GEORGII and his colleagues did not test for the presence of the virus immediately, but grew the embryo tissue in culture for 3 days or more before testing for the presence of virus. This would probably be a less sensitive test than the direct method.

CRISPENS (1967a) found that females infected between 0 and 9 days before conception were more likely to have infected offspring than mice infected 10 or more days before conception. CRISPENS (1967b) also observed that among the weanlings born to mothers infected with LDV between 10 and 19 days before conception there were more females (male:female ratio 40.6:59.4) than expected. In litters born to uninfected females and females infected 0 to 9 and 20 to 29 days before conception the ratio was approximately 50:50. To determine if the infection was acting via one or both parents, CRISPENS (1969) infected male and female mice with LDV 10 days before mating them with normal non-infected mice. The sex ratio among the offspring of infected females mated to control males was identical to that observed in control mice (51:49) but with the control females mated to infected males the ratio was 43:57. It is clear that the virus is acting on the male parent and it is interesting that none of the offspring were infected in the male infected group. The injection of male mice with mouse liver LDH, 20,000 units at daily intervals for 8 days before mating with uninfected females, resulted in offspring with a sex ratio 45:55 as compared to 51:49 for the control mice. The difference is not significant but it must be remembered that the level of injected enzyme would fall rapidly after injection and so it can not be assumed that the effect on the sex ratio is not due to the high level of LDH in infected mice. These results were obtained using C57BL/Fg mice. Using BALB/cDg mice which have a low male:female sex ratio CRISPENS (1971) found that if females were injected with virus 10 to 14 days before mating the litters contained more males than expected (males:females ratio 49:51 as compared to 41:59 in the controls). CRISPENS found that plasma LDH levels were very similar in LDV-infected C57BL/Fg and BALB/cDg mice but that spermatozoa LDH levels in samples from non-infected BALB/cDg mice were higher than in LDV-infected mice, whereas the levels in infected and non-infected C57BL/Fg mice were similar.

There is only one report of a foster nursing experiment. CRISPENS (1964b) fostered 3 litters from uninfected females onto 3 females infected one week previously and one litter from an infected female onto a normal mouse. On examination, when five weeks old, none of the young were infected.

The male appears to play no part in the transmission of the infection to the young and when normal female mice are mated with infected males for 11 days, only 2 of the 9 exposed females became infected (ROWSON, 1962).

As the LDH virus is not readily transmitted from parents to young, the maintenance of the infection depends on transmission of the virus between adults. Infected food and environment are likely to play a part in this but as the infection is rare in laboratory stock mice, although the virus is accidentally maintained in many laboratories by experimental procedures, it seems unlikely that cross infection, on any significant scale, occurs by transmission of excreta between mice. The maintenance of the virus in the wild therefore probably depends on transmission during fighting and cannibalism, which is probably frequent but the role of blood sucking parasites should not be dismissed. Since LDV-infected mice have a permanent viraemia, transmission of the virus by insects or mites could be an important means of maintaining the infection in wild mouse populations. No studies of the ability of the virus to infect parasitic vectors have been reported, however. It would be interesting to know which blood-sucking parasites are able to transmit LDV and for how long they remain infectious after a blood meal.

# VIII. Laboratory Methods

## A. Blood Samples from Mice for LDH Estimation

Mouse blood haemolyses very readily, thus it is very difficult to obtain serum free of all haemolysis and suitable for LDH estimations. It is therefore much easier to use plasma. Mice may be bled from the brachial artery, the tail (ADAMS, ROWSON, and SALAMAN, 1961) or retro-orbital sinus (SALEM, GROSSMANN, and BILBEY, 1963; RILEY, 1960) but whichever method is used there must be a minimum of tissue damage. Bleeding from the retro-orbital sinus is easily performed under ether anaesthesia and is the method of choice for most purposes but if the mouse is to be bled repeatedly at frequent intervals the LDH activity in the plasma may be found to rise slightly presumably due to tissue damage. For repeated sampling tail bleeding is more satisfactory but the mouse should be kept at 37° C for 10 minutes before bleeding and the minimum of pressure applied to the tail after the tip has been cut off cleanly with sharp scissors. If a larger volume of blood is required the brachial artery is the best site. Under ether anaesthesia a mid-line incision is made and the tissues reflected. If the skin is held up the axilla forms a pocket into which the blood will flow when the brachial artery is cut. A drop of heparin is placed in the axilla before the artery is cut and the freely flowing blood taken up with a pipette. Care must be taken to cause the minimum of tissue damage as this will produce an abnormally high LDH level. The blood should be taken into a heparinized tube or diluted in phosphate buffered saline containing 100 I. U. per ml of heparin without preservative. The blood, appropriately diluted, should be centrifuged at 2,000$g$ for 10 minutes and the dilute plasma carefully removed. It is advisable to remove only the upper three quarters of the plasma so as to avoid any contamination with cells. Plasma LDH activity is quite stable and plasma samples can be kept overnight at +4° C without appreciable loss of activity but for longer storage the plasma should be frozen (CRISPENS, 1962).

## B. Estimation of Plasma LDH Activity

### 1. Quantitative Methods

Lactic dehydrogenase converts lactate to pyruvate and in the process nicotin-amide-adenine dinucleotide (NAD) is reduced:

$$\text{L-lactate} + \text{NAD}^+ \rightleftharpoons \text{pyruvate} + \text{NADH}$$

The activity of the enzyme can be assayed in the forward reaction by measuring the increase in NADH or in the backward reaction (using pyruvate as substrate) by measuring the disappearance of pyruvate or NADH. A method involving the change in NADH concentration is the most accurate and the change in NADH concentration is easily followed by measuring the absorption change at 340 nm. However, if a spectrophotometer is not available the method measuring the fall in pyruvate concentration may be useful.

*a) Determination of Plasma LDH by Spectrophotometric Method*
(Backward Reaction) (WRÓBLEWSKI and LA DUE, 1955).

*Principle*

$$\text{Pyruvate} + \text{NADH} \xrightarrow[\text{LDH}]{} \text{Lactate} + \text{NAD}^+$$

Plasma is incubated with pyruvate and NADH at 25° C, and the resultant decrease in optical density due to the oxidation of NADH is measured at 340 nm. The rate of the reaction is proportional to the amount of LDH present.

*Reagents*

*Phosphate Buffer*, pH 7.4

13.97 g di-potassium hydrogen phosphate (anhydrous). 2.69 g potassium dihydrogen phosphate (anhydrous). Dissolve in distilled water, make up to 1 litre and store in the cold.

*NADH*, 2.5 mg/ml
  Weigh accurately 10 mg reduced nicotinamide adenine dinucleotide in a 5 ml bijou bottle. Add exactly 4 ml phosphate buffer.
  Store frozen for not more than 2 days.

*Sodium Pyruvate*, 2.5 mg/ml
  Weigh accurately 10 mg sodium pyruvate in a 5 ml bijou bottle.
  Add exactly 4 ml phosphate buffer and store frozen.

*Method*
  Pipette into a 1 cm cell:
Buffer — 2.6 ml.
Diluted plasma (1 in 6) — 0.2 ml.
NADH — 0.1 ml.
Stand for 15 minutes then add pyruvate — 0.1 ml.
Follow the decrease in optical density at 340 nm for 6 minutes (*e.g.* read at 0, 1, 2, 3, 4, 5 and 6 minutes).

*Calculation*
  One conventional (spectrophotometric) unit of LDH activity produces a decrease in optical density of 0.001 per minute per ml plasma. Thus, using 0.2 ml plasma under the above conditions the change in optical density calculated for a 5 minute period, multiplied by 1,000, and multiplied by the plasma dilution employed, *i.e.* 6, will give the plasma LDH activity in conventional units. The reaction temperature should be within 24° to 27° C.

## b) Determination of Plasma LDH by Spectrophotometric Method

(Forward Reaction) (AMADOR, DORFMAN and WACKER, 1963).

*Principle*

$$\text{Lactate} + \text{NAD}^+ \xrightarrow[\text{LDH}]{} \text{Pyruvate} + \text{NADH}$$

  Plasma is incubated with lactate and $NAD^+$ at 25° C, and the resultant increase in optical density due to the reduction of NAD is measured at 340 nm. The rate of reaction is proportional to the amount of LDH present over a wide range; the reaction is linear over a wider range of activities than is the backward reaction (AMADOR, DORFMAN, and WACKER, 1963).

*Reagents*
  Buffered solution of lactic acid (77.5 mM), sodium pyrophosphate (0.05 M, pH 8.8) and NAD (5.25 mM). Dissolve 6.2 g sodium pyrophosphate in 250 ml hot distilled water, cool, add lactic acid (2.0 ml) and adjust to pH 8.8 with 1 N sodium hydroxide. Dissolve 1.10 g NAD in this solution and adjust to 280 ml. Then store in 2.8 ml aliquots at —20° C. These reaction mixtures are stable for 6 months.

*Method*
  Pipette into a 1 cm cell:
Reaction mixture    2.8 ml
Plasma              0.2 ml
  Mix well by inversion and follow the increase in optical density at 340 nm every minute for six minutes. If the reaction rate exceeds a change in absorbance of 0.100 per minute, the plasma should be diluted.

*Calculation*
  Under the above conditions, the change in optical density calculated from a 5 minute period and multiplied by 1,000 and by the plasma dilution employed will give the plasma LDH activity in conventional units. The reaction temperature should be within 24° to 27° C.

## c) Determination of Plasma LDH by Colorimetric Method
### (Disappearance of Pyruvate)

The method is fully described in Sigma technical bulletin No. 500. It is not so accurate or reliable as the previous two methods (AMADOR, REINSTEIN, and BEN-NOTTI, 1965), but can be of value where a spectrophotometer measuring absorption at 340 nm is not available.

### Principle

A standard amount of sodium pyruvate and excess NADH are incubated with 0.1 ml of diluted serum for 30 minutes after which a colour reagent is added which gives a brown colour with the unchanged pyruvate. The intensity of the brown colour gives a measure of the amount of pyruvate remaining unaltered by the enzyme.

### Reagents

*NADH and Pyruvate Substrate.* 1 mg NADH (Boehringer) per ml of standard pyruvate substrate (Sigma). The pyruvate substrate provided by Sigma gives satisfactory results but other preparations of pyruvate may not.

#### Colour Reagent

200 mg 2:4 dinitrophenylhydrazine dissolved in 85 ml concentrated hydrochloric acid and diluted to 1 litre. It may be stored at $+4°$ C in the dark.

*0.4 N Sodium Hydroxide* preferably carbon dioxide free.

### Method

*Preparation of Calibration Curve.* Into 6 test tubes place 1.0, 0.8, 0.6, 0.4, 0.2 and 0.1 ml of Sigma pyruvate substrate and 0.1, 0.3, 0.5, 0.7, 0.9 and 1.0 ml of water so that the total volume in each tube is 1.1 ml. To each tube add 1 ml of colour reagent. Mix gently and leave at 25° C ($±5°$ C) for 20 minutes. Add to each tube 10 ml of 0.4 N sodium hydroxide. Wait at least 5 minutes but not more than 30 minutes. Then read optical density or per cent transmission for each tube using water as reference. A wave length or filter system should be used which will give an optical density of 0.9 (12 per cent transmission) for tube No. 1 (1.0 ml pyruvate substrate). The same wave length or filter system must be used in all subsequent tests. With these data a standard curve can be prepared: tube 1 represents no enzyme activity, tube 2 280 u, tube 3 640 u, tube 4 1,040 u, tube 5 1,530 u and tube 6 2,000 u.

*Estimation of LDH Activity.* Pipette 1 ml of NADH pyruvate substrate into as many tubes as there are sera to be tested. Place the tubes in a 37° C water bath for a few minutes to warm. Add 0.1 ml of test serum diluted 1 in 6 with water, shake the tube gently and start a timer. Add the other sera at 30 second intervals to the other tubes. Exactly 30 minutes after adding the sera remove the tubes from the water bath and add 1,0 ml of colour reagent. After 20 minutes add 10.0 ml of 0.4 N sodium hydroxide to each tube. Wait 5 minutes but not more than 30 minutes before reading the optical density under the conditions used for the calibration curve. Determine the LDH activity from the calibration curve.

## 2. Qualitative Method

### Principal

1. Pyruvate + reduced nicotinamide-adenine dinucleotide

$$(\text{NADH}) \xrightarrow[\text{LDH}]{} \text{Lactate} + \text{NAD}$$

2. Pyruvate + 2:4 dinitrophenylhydrazine → Pyruvate-dinitrophenylhydrazone.

LDH catalyzes reaction 1, the rate of reaction being proportional to the amount of LDH present. Plasma is incubated at 37° C with pyruvate and NADH, and the pyruvate remaining after reaction is demonstrated by addition of 2:4 dinitrophenylhydrazine, which forms an intensely brown coloured hydrazone in presence of pyruvate and NaOH. In the following test, the amounts of the various reagents have been so adjusted that plasmas having an LDH activity of 1500 I.U./ml or more will consume all the pyruvate present during the first incubation, resulting in a colourless mixture. Plasmas with a low LDH activity, less than 1000 I.U./ml, show up with a brown colour. The method is thus ideally suited for titrating LDV.

*Reagents*

*NADH-Pyruvate Substrate.* 1 mg NADH (DPNH) (Boehringer) per millilitre standardized pyruvate substrate (Sigma No. 500L-1).

*Colour Reagent*
200 mg 2:4 dinitrophenylhydrazine.
85 ml conc. HCl.
Diluate to 1 litre and store at +4° C in the dark
2 N *Sodium Hydroxide* (preferably $CO_2$ free).
*Control Plasma.* Plasma from a high LDH mouse, diluted to 100 I.U. LDH/ml.

*Method*

Warm 'spot plate' (haemagglutination tray) in 37° C incubator.

Pipette 0.1 ml NADH-pyruvate substrate into each depression (plan on one depression per test plus two for controls).

Add 0.05 ml of plasma diluted 1 in 24 at timed intervals (say quarter-minute), with stirring. Include one 'blank' depression and one with control plasma. Incubate at 37° C for 30 minutes.

Exactly 30 minutes after adding the diluted plasma, add 0.1 ml colour reagent to each depression with stirring.

Incubate 10 minutes at room temperature.

Pipette 0.2 ml 2 N NaOH into each depression, with stirring.

Read immediately — high LDH — colourless; low LDH — brown (a typical result is presented in Fig. 7, page 14).

*Summary*

|                 | Test | Reagent Control | Test Control |
|-----------------|------|-----------------|--------------|
| NADH-Pyruvate   | 0.1  | 0.1             | 0.1          |
| 1/24 Plasma     | 0.5  | —               | —            |
| Control plasma  | —    | —               | 0.05         |
| Colour Reagent  | 0.1  | 0.1             | 0.1          |
| 2 N NaOH        | 0.2  | 0.2             | 0.2          |

## 3. Units of LDH Activity (KING and MOSS, 1963)

One conventional unit of LDH activity is the amount of enzyme which will catalyze the oxidation of NADH to NAD causing a decrease in optical density at 340 nm of 0.001 optical density per minute at 25° C. The conventional unit derived from simple observed changes in optical density can be converted to the more universal basis of substrate utilization.

1 conventional unit causes a decrease of optical density at 340 nm of 0.001/min/cm. Since 1 micromole of NADH in 1 ml of solution has an optical density of 6.3/cm at 340 nm, 1 micromole of NADH will have an optical density of 2.1 in the 3 ml reaction mixture.

1 conventional unit $= 0.001/2.1$ micromoles of NADH reduced per minute
$= 0.00048$ micromoles of NADH reduced per minute
approximately $0.0005$ micromoles of NADH reduced per minute

1 conventional unit/ml $= 0.0005$ micromoles/minute/ml
$= 0.5$ micromoles/minute/liter
$= 0.5$ international unit

Since the Commission on Enzymes defines a Standard unit as the amount of an enzyme which will catalyze the transformation of one micromole of the substrate per minute under defined conditions and the concentration of an enzyme in solution should be expressed as units per ml, 1 conventional unit $= 0.0005$ Standard units. As this definition requires dividing the observed conventional units by 200 it brings all normal values below unity. This can be avoided by using the Commission's recommended term milli-unit, which makes them identical with the International units. The same may be accomplished by expressing the activity in terms of millimicromoles of NADH.

1 conventional unit $= 0.5$ International unit (KING and CAMPBELL, 1961)
$= 0.0005$ Standard unit (Commission on Enzymes, 1961)
$= 0.5$ Standard milliunit (Commission on Enzymes, 1961)

## C. Diagnosis of LDV Infection in Mice

Laboratory stock mice are seldom infected with LDV and the absence of infection can be confirmed by demonstrating that their plasma LDH level is below 500 I.U. per ml. Except for the first 48 hours after infection, infected mice always have a plasma LDH level above 500 I.U. per ml. If a mouse has a raised plasma LDH level the presence of an infective agent can be proved by taking blood or any other tissue and injecting this into a normal mouse. The test mouse is bled from the orbit after 3 days for plasma LDH level. If the mouse appears healthy and has a raised LDH level the presence of LDH virus is virtually certain, but to exclude the possibility of *Eperythrozoon coccoides* being the cause of the elevated LDH level the titre of the infective agent in the plasma 24 hours after infection should be determined. A titre of $10^8$ infective doses per ml of plasma excludes the possibility of other agents than LDV. Alternatively *Eperythrozoon coccoides* may be directly excluded by injecting material into a group of splenectomized mice and examining blood films from them 2, 4, 6, 8 and 10 days after injection for the organisms.

## D. Virus Titration

Tenfold dilutions are prepared in phosphate buffered saline with 10 per cent broth and 0.2 ml volumes injected intravenously (orbital sinus) or intraperitoneally into groups of mice. Ideally the mice should be housed in individual cages but as LDV is not rapidly transmitted between mice the mice receiving each dose level may be kept in the same cage. After 72 hours the mice are bled from the orbit and a qualitative test for LDH activity performed on the plasma. A sharp endpoint is usually obtained and the virus titre estimated by Thompson's method (THOMPSON, 1947).

# References

ADAMS, D. H., and B. M. BOWMAN: An anti-virus action of azaserine-thioguanine *in vivo*. Nature (Lond.) **197**, 316—317 (1963).

ADAMS, D. H., and B. M. BOWMAN: Studies on the properties of factors elevating the activity of mouse-plasma lactate dehydrogenase. Biochem. J. **90**, 477—482 (1964).

ADAMS, D. H., and E. J. FIELD: A plasma lactic dehydrogenase-elevating virus associated with scrapie-infected mice. J. gen. Virol. **1**, 449—454 (1967).

ADAMS, D. H., K. E. K. ROWSON, and M. H. SALAMAN: The effect of tumours, of leukaemia, and of some viruses associated with them, on the plasma lactic dehydrogenase activity of mice. Brit. J. Cancer **15**, 860—867 (1961).

ALLISON, A. C.: Interference and interferon in relation to tumor viruses and tumor cells. In: Viruses, Nucleic Acids, and Cancer, pp. 462—484. Baltimore: Williams & Wilkins Co., 1963.

ALMEIDA, J. D., D. M. BERRY, C. H. CUNNINGHAM, D. HAMRE, M. S. HOFSTAD, L. MALLUCCI, K. MCINTOSH, and D. A. J. TYRRELL: Coronaviruses. Nature (Lond.) **220**, 650 (1968).

ALMEIDA, J. D., and C. A. MIMS: The unique morphology of the lactic dehydrogenase agent. Microbios **10**, 175—180 (1974).

ALMEIDA, J. D., and A. P. WATERSON: The morphology of virus-antibody interaction. Advanc. Virus Res. **15**, 307—338 (1969).

AMADOR, E., L. E. DORFMAN, and W. E. C. WACKER: Serum lactic dehydrogenase activity; analytical assessment of current assays. Clin. Chem. **9**, 391—399 (1963).

AMADOR, E., H. REINSTEIN, and N. BENOTTI: Precision and accuracy of lactic dehydrogenase assays. Amer. J. clin. Path. **44**, 62—70 (1965).

ANDERSON, S. G., and G. L. ADA: Murray valley encephalitis virus: preparation of an infective "ribonucleic acid" fraction. Aust. J. exp. Biol. med. Sci. **37**, 353—364 (1959).

ANDERSON, H. C., V. RILEY, M. A. FITZMAURICE, J. D. LOVELESS, P. WADE, and A. E. MOORE: Quantitative study of the lactate dehydrogenase-elevating virus in mouse embryo cultures. J. nat. Cancer Inst. **36**, 89—95 (1966).

ANDERSON, H. C., V. RILEY, P. WADE, and A. E. MOORE: Quantitative evidence for propagation of the lactate dehydrogenase (LDH) elevating virus in mouse embryo cell cultures. Proc. Amer. Ass. Cancer Res. **6**, 2 (1965).

ANDREWES, C. H., D. BLASKOVIC, J. B. BROOKSBY, J. CASALS, H. S. GINSBERG, M. M. KAPLAN, J. MAURIN, J. L. MELNICK, H. G. PEREIRA, R. ROTT, P. TOURNIER, C. J. YORK, and V. ZHDANOV: Generic names of viruses of vertebrates. Virology **40**, 1070—1071 (1970).

ANDREWES, C. H., and D. M. HORSTMANN: The susceptibility of viruses to ethyl ether. J. gen. Microbiol. **3**, 290—297 (1949).

ANDREWES, C. H., and H. G. PEREIRA: Viruses of Vertebrates, 3rd Ed. London: Baillière Tindall, 1972.

ANSARI, K. A., C. F. NEILSON, and P. G. STANSLY: Pathogenesis of infectious splenic enlargement in mice. Exp. molec. Path. **2**, 61—68 (1963).

ARISON, R. N., J. A. CASSARO, and C. E. SHONK: Factors which affect plasma lactic dehydrogenase in tumor-bearing mice. Proc. Soc. exp. Biol. (N.Y.) **113**, 497—501 (1963).

ASADA, M., and J. T. GALAMBOS: Sorbitol dehydrogenase and hepatocellular injury: an experimental and clinical study. Gastroenterology **44**, 578—587 (1963).

ASHE, W. K., and A. L. NOTKINS: Neutralization of an infectious herpes simplex virus-antibody complex by anti-γ-globulin. Proc. nat. Acad. Sci. (Wash.) **56**, 447—451 (1966).

ASHERSON, G. L., and M. BENDINELLI: Immunodepression by viruses: effect of Friend and Riley viruses on contact sensitivity. G. Microbiol. **17**, 179—188 (1969).

BAILEY, J. M., J. CLOUGH, and A. LOHAUS: Influence of LDH virus on growth of Ehrlich ascites tumor in mice. Proc. Soc. exp. Biol. (N.Y.) **119**, 1200—1204 (1965).

BAILEY, J. M., J. CLOUGH, A. LOHAUS, and D. A. WRIGHT: A comparative study of LDH viruses from different tumors. Fed. Proc. **24**, 597 (1965).

BAILEY, J. M., J. CLOUGH, and M. STEARMAN: Plasma enzymes erythropoiesis and R.E.S. function in mice following infection with an LDH agent. Proc. Soc. exp. Biol. (N.Y.) **115**, 642—646 (1964a).

BAILEY, J. M., J. CLOUGH, and M. STEARMAN: Clearance of plasma enzymes in normal and LDH agent-infected mice. Proc. Soc. exp. Biol. (N.Y.) **117**, 350—354 (1964b).

BAILEY, J. M., and M. MONROE: Studies on replication of LDH virus. Fed. Proc. **31**, 836 (1972).

BAILEY, J. M., M. STEARMAN, and J. CLOUGH: LDH levels in blood and tissues of mice infected with LDH agent. Proc. Soc. exp. Biol. (N.Y.) **114**, 148—153 (1963).

BAILEY, J. M., and D. A. WRIGHT: Plasma enzyme elevations with LDH viruses from different tumors. Proc. Soc. exp. Biol. (N.Y.) **120**, 346—350 (1965).

BALTIMORE, D.: Expression of animal virus genomes. Bact. Rev. **35**, 235—241 (1971).

BARON, S., C. E. BUCKLER, R. M. FRIEDMAN, and R. V. McCLOSKEY: Role of interferon during viraemia in mice. Bact. Proc. p. 116 (1964).

BARON, S., C. E. BUCKLER, R. V. McCLOSKEY, and R. L. KIRSCHSTEIN: Role of interferon during viraemia. 1. Production of circulating interferon. J. Immunol. **96**, 12—16 (1966).

BARON, S., H. G. DU BUY, C. E. BUCKLER, and M. L. JOHNSON: Relationship of interferon production to virus growth *in vivo*. Proc. Soc. exp. Biol. (N.Y.) **117**, 338—341 (1964).

BAYERLE, H., A. GEORGII und P. JAKOB: Über das Verhalten des Lactatdehydrogenase aktivierenden Virus aus Mäusegeschwülsten bei der Autolyse. Z. Krebsforsch. **65**, 171—172 (1962).

BAYERLE, H., A. GEORGII und K. E. RICHARD: Über die Aktivität von Serumfermenten nach zellfreier Beimpfung mit Ehrlich'schem Mäusetumorascites. Klin. Wschr. **40**, 920 (1962).

BELL, R. L.: Separation of serum lactic dehydrogenase originating in myocardial and hepatic tissue, by means of heat fractionation. Amer. J. clin. Path. **40**, 216—221 (1963).

BENDINELLI, M.: Conoscenze attuali sul virus di Riley o virus LDH. Ann. Sclavo **9**, 253—280 (1967).

BENDINELLI, M., and G. L. ASHERSON: Depression of contact sensitivity by Friend and Riley viruses. Boll. Ist. sieroter. milan. **50**, 502—507 (1971).

BIERMAN, H. R., B. R. HILL, L. REINHARDT, and E. EMORY: Correlation of serum lactic dehydrogenase activity with the clinical status of patients with cancer, lymphomas and the leukemias. Cancer Res. **17**, 660—667 (1957).

BILBEY, D. L. J., and T. NICOL: Effect of various natural steroids on the phagocytic activity of the reticuloendothelial system. Nature (Lond.) **182**, 674 (1958).

BLADEN, H. A., and A. L. NOTKINS: Electron microscopic demonstration of the lactic dehydrogenase agent. Virology **21**, 269—271 (1963).

BORDEN, E. C., R. E. SHOPE, and F. A. MURPHY: Physicochemical and morphological relationships of some arthropod-borne viruses to Bluetongue virus — A new taxonomic group. Physicochemical and serological studies. J. gen. Virol. **13**, 261—271 (1971).

BOYD, J. W.: The rates of disappearance of L-lactate dehydrogenase isoenzymes from plasma. Biochim. biophys. Acta (Amst.) **132**, 221—231 (1967a).

BOYD, J. W.: The disappearance of $^{14}$C-labelled isoenzyme 5 of L-lactate dehydrogenase. Biochim. biophys. Acta (Amst.) **146**, 590—593 (1967b).

BOYD, J. W., and A. W. PHILLIPS: Inhibition of Lymphoma 6C3 HED by L-asparaginase from *Serratia marcescens*. J. nat. Cancer Inst. **46**, 1271—1276 (1971).

BRDICZKA, D., A. GEORGII und H. ZOBL: Die Wirkung von Nucleinsäuren aus virushaltigen Mäusegeschwulsten auf die Lactatdehydrogenaseaktivität in Blutserum. Naturwissenschaften **50**, 306—307 (1963).

BRIER, A. M., C. WOHLENBERG, J. ROSENTHAL, M. MAGE, and A. L. NOTKINS: Inhibition or enhancement of immunological injury of virus infected cells. Proc. nat. Acad. Sci. (Wash.) **68**, 3073—3077 (1971).

BROOME, J. D.: Factors which may influence the effectiveness of L-asparaginases as tumor inhibitors. Brit. J. Cancer **22**, 595—602 (1968).

BROOME, J. D.: Antilymphoma activity of L-asparaginase *in vivo:* clearance rates of enzyme preparations from guinea pig serum and yeast in relation to their effect on tumor growth. J. nat. Cancer Inst. **35**, 967—974 (1965).

BRUNNER, K. T., D. HUREZ, R. T. McCLOSKEY, and B. BENACERRAF: Blood clearance of $P^{32}$-labelled vesicular stomatitis and Newcastle disease viruses by the reticulo-endothelial system in mice. J. Immunol. **85**, 99—105 (1960).

BURGESS, E. A., and G. SYLVÉN: Lactic dehydrogenase activity in plasma and interstitial fluid during growth of mouse tumors. Cancer Res. **23**, 714—719 (1963).

BUSCHER, T. J., C. FRANTSI, and K. F. GREGORY: Fluctuating virus and enzyme levels in plasma of mice infected with Friend leukemia virus. Canad. J. Microbiol. **17**, 315—321 (1971).

CAHN, R. D., N. O. KAPLAN, L. LEVINE, and E. ZWILLING: Nature and development of lactic dehydrogenase. Science **136**, 962—969 (1962).

CARVER, D. H.: Personal communication (1969).

CARVER, D. H., P. I. MARCUS, and D. S. Y. SETO: Intrinsic interference: a unique interference system used in assaying non-cytopathic viruses. Arch. ges. Virusforsch. **22**, 55—60 (1967).

CASSELS, A. C.: The release of lactate dehydrogenase from chick embryo cells infected with Semliki Forest virus. J. gen. Virol. **18**, 203—205 (1973).

CHENG, P.-Y.: Infectivity of ribonucleic acid from mouse brains infected with Semliki forest virus. Nature (Lond.) **181**, 1800 (1958).

CLOUGH, J. D., and J. M. BAILEY: Mechanism of plasma enzyme elevation by tumor LDH agent. Tex. Rep. Biol. Med. **23**, 644—645 (1965).

Commission on enzymes: Report International Union of Biochemistry. New York: Macmillan (Pergamon), 1961.

CONGDON, C. C.: Lymphatic tissue germinal centers in immune reactions. Progr. Biophys. molec. Biol. **19**, 308—337 (1969). Oxford, England: Pergamon Press Ltd., 1969.

CRISPENS, C. G.: Effect of storage on serum lactic dehydrogenase activity. Amer. Zool. **2**, 515—516 (1962).

CRISPENS, C. G.: Serum lactic dehydrogenase levels in mice during the development of autochthonous and chemically induced tumors. J. nat. Cancer Inst. **30**, 361—366 (1963a).

CRISPENS, C. G.: A lactic dehydrogenase elevating agent in association with human neoplasms. Nature (Lond.) **199**, 1202—1203 (1963b).

CRISPENS, C. G.: Factors which influence normal values for serum lactic dehydrogenase in mice. Experientia (Basel) **19**, 97—98 (1963c).

CRISPENS, C. G.: A preliminary report on attempts to demonstrate virus like entities in association with human neoplasms. Anat. Rec. **145**, 314 (1963d).

CRISPENS, C. G.: Preliminary studies on in utero transmission of the lactic dehydrogenase agent. Anat. Res. **149**, 511 (1964a).

CRISPENS, C. G.: On the epizootiology of the lactic dehydrogenase agent. J. nat. Cancer Inst. **32**, 497—505 (1964b).

CRISPENS, C. G.: Mouse plasma lactic dehydrogenase elevation: evidence for two particles. Virology **24**, 501—502 (1964c).

CRISPENS, C. G.: The lactic dehydrogenase agent; its possible implications for the virologist and the oncologist. Bull. Sch. Med. Maryland **49**, vii (1964d).

CRISPENS, C. G.: On the properties of the lactic dehydrogenase agent. J. nat. Cancer Inst. **35**, 975—979 (1965a).

CRISPENS, C. G.: On the transmission of the lactic dehydrogenase agent from mother to offspring. J. nat. Cancer Inst. **34**, 331—336 (1965b).

CRISPENS, C. G.: Properties of lactic dehydrogenase elevating agents. Anat. Rec. **151**, 448—449 (1965c).

CRISPENS, C. G.: Effect of actinomycin D on mice infected with lactate dehydrogenase virus. Experientia (Basel) **22**, 823—824 (1966a).

CRISPENS, C. G.: Effect of thymectomy on mice infected with the lactate dehydrogenase agent. J. nat. Cancer Inst. **36**, 81—87 (1966b).

CRISPENS, C. G.: Association of the lactate dehydrogenase virus (Riley) with chemically induced murine neoplasms. Anat. Rec. **154**, 456—457 (1966c).

CRISPENS, C. G.: Lactate dehydrogenase virus and mouse embryos. Nature (Lond.) **214**, 819 (1967a).

CRISPENS, C. G.: The lactate dehydrogenase virus: variations in the sex ratio of weanling mice. Anat. Rec. **157**, 232 (1967b).

CRISPENS, C. G.: Antibody response in normal and neonatally thymectomized mice infected with the lactate dehydrogenase virus. Anat. Rec. **160**, 466 (1968).

CRISPENS, C. G.: Additional studies on the effect of the lactate dehydrogenase virus on murine sex ratios. Experientia (Basel) **25**, 1197—1198 (1969).

CRISPENS, C. G.: Effect of statolon on lactate dehydrogenase virus infection in mice. Arch. ges. Virusforsch. **31**, 191—195 (1970a).

CRISPENS, C. G.: Lactate dehydrogenase virus association with transplantable murine tumors. Experientia (Basel) **26**, 891—892 (1970b).

CRISPENS, C. G.: Effect of the lactate dehydrogenase virus on the incidence of lymphocytic leukemia in $C_3H/Fg$ mice. Anat. Rec. **166**, 294 (1970c).

CRISPENS, C. G.: Studies on the response of SJL/J mice to infection with the lactate dehydrogenase virus. Arch. ges. Virusforsch. **35**, 177—182 (1971).

CRISPENS, C. G.: Genetic control of the response of SJL/J mice to LDH virus infection. Arch. ges. Virusforsch. **38**, 225—227 (1972).

CRISPENS, C. G., and T. A. BURNS: Electronmicroscope investigation of lactic dehydrogenase agent. Nature (Lond.) **204**, 1302 (1964).

CRISPENS, C. G., and I. F. REY: Additional studies on the effect of neonatal thymectomy and lactate dehydrogenase virus infection on mice. Experientia (Basel) **23**, 681—683 (1967).

CRISPENS, C. G., and W. K. WHITTEN: Strain differences in sex ratio response of mice to lactate dehydrogenase virus infection. Experientia (Basel) **27**, 41—42 (1971).

DALTON, A. J., F. HAGUENAU, and J. B. MOLONEY: Morphology of particles associated with murine leukemia as revealed by negative staining: preliminary report. J. nat. Cancer Inst. **29**, 1177—1178 (1962).

DARNELL, M. B., and P. G. W. PLAGEMANN: Physical properties of lactic dehydrogenase-elevating virus and its ribonucleic acid. J. Virol. **10**, 1082—1085 (1972).

DARNELL, M. B., and P. G. W. PLAGEMANN: Replication of lactic dehydrogenase-elevating virus and its ribonucleic acid in peritoneal macrophage cultures. Abstr. ann. Meet. Amer. Soc. Microbiol., p. 203 (1973).

DE HARVEN, E.: Viraemia in Friend murine leukemia: the electron microscope approach to the problem. Path. et Biol. **13**, 125—134 (1965).

DE HARVEN, E., and C. FRIEND: Structure of virus particles partially purified from the blood of leukemic mice. Virology **23**, 119—124 (1964).

DE HARVEN, E., and C. FRIEND: Origin of the viremia in murine leukemia. Nat. Cancer Inst. Monogr. No. **22**, 79—105 (1966).

DENT, P. B.: Immunodepression by oncogenic viruses. Progr. med. Virol. **14**, 1—35 (1972).

DE THÉ, G., and A. L. NOTKINS: Ultrastructure of the lactic dehydrogenase virus (LDV) and cell-virus relationships. Virology **26**, 512—516 (1965).

DIMMOCK, N. J., and D. A. J. TYRRELL: Some physico-chemical properties of rhinoviruses. Brit. J. exp. Path. **45**, 271—280 (1964).

DREYFUS, J.-CL., G. SCHAPIRA et J. DEMOS: Étude de la créatine-kinase sérique chez les myopathes et leurs familles. Rev. franç. Étud. clin. biol. **5**, 384—386 (1960).

DREYFUS, J. C., G. SCHAPIRA, and F. SCHAPIRA: Serum enzymes in the physiopathology of muscle. Ann. N.Y. Acad. Sci. **75**, 235—249 (1958).

DU BUY, H., S. BARON, C. UHLENDORF, and M. L. JOHNSON: Role of interferon in murine lactic dehydrogenase virus infection, *in vivo* and *in vitro*. Infection and Immunity **8**, 977—984 (1973).

DU BUY, H. G., and M. L. JOHNSON: Some properties of the lactic dehydrogenase agent of mice. J. exp. Med. **122**, 587—600 (1965).

DU BUY, H. G., and M. L. JOHNSON: Studies on the *in vitro* and *in vivo* multiplication of the LDH virus of mice. J. exp. Med. **123**, 985—998 (1966).

Du Buy, H. G., and M. L. Johnson: Further studies on the *in vitro* replication of lactic dehydrogenase virus in peritoneal macrophage cultures. Proc. Soc. exp. Biol. (N.Y.) **128**, 1210—1214 (1968).

Du Buy, H. G., and M. L. Johnson: Effect of actinomycin D on lactic dehydrogenase virus multiplication in mouse macrophages. Proc. Soc. exp. Biol. (N.Y.) **133**, 1023 to 1025 (1970).

Du Buy, H. G., M. Worthington, and M. L. Johnson: Effect of an immunosuppressive agent, cyclophosphamide on chronic lactic dehydrogenase virus viremia of mice. Infection and Immunity **4**, 720—724 (1971).

Ebert, P. S., M. A. Chirigos, and S. P. Chan: Studies on the enzymology of the rhabdomyosarcoma induced by the murine sarcoma virus (Moloney). Cancer Res. **30**, 960—965 (1970).

Ebert, P. S., M. A. Chirigos, and P. A. Ellsworth: Differential response of Friend leukemia virus and lactate dehydrogenase virus to chemotherapy and *in vitro* neutralization. Cancer Res. **28**, 363—367 (1968).

Ebert, P. S., M. A. Chirigos, L. A. Fields, and P. A. Ellsworth: Plasma lactate dehydrogenase and spleen heme biosynthetic activity following Friend and Rauscher leukemia virus infections. Life Sci. **6**, 1963—1971 (1967).

Elliott, B. A., E. M. Jepson, and J. H. Wilkinson: Serum α-hydroxybutyrate dehydrogenase — A new test with improved specificity for myocardial lesions. Clin. Sci. **23**, 305—316 (1962).

Elliott, B. A., and J. H. Wilkinson: The serum "α-hydroxybutyrate dehydrogenase" in diseases other than myocardial infarction. Clin. Sci. **24**, 343—355 (1963).

Evans, R.: Replication of Riley's plasma enzyme elevating virus *in vitro*. J. gen. Microbiol. **37**, vii (1964).

Evans, R.: Replication of Riley's plasma enzymes-elevating virus in tissue culture: the importance of the cellular composition. J. gen. Virol. **1**, 363—374 (1967).

Evans, R.: Factors affecting replication of the lactate dehydrogenase-elevating virus (LDH virus) in peritoneal macrophage. J. gen. Microbiol. **57**, XXI (1969).

Evans, R.: Further studies on the replication of the lactate dehydrogenase-elevating virus (LDH virus) in mouse peritoneal macrophage cultures. Proc. Soc. exp. Biol. (N.Y.) **133**, 831—836 (1970).

Evans, R., and V. Riley: Circulating interferon in mice infected with the lactate dehydrogenase-elevating virus. J. gen. Virol. **3**, 449—452 (1968).

Evans, R., and M. H. Salaman: Studies on the mechanism of action of Riley virus. III. Replication of Riley's plasma enzyme-elevating virus *in vitro*. J. exp. Med. **122**, 993—1002 (1965).

Falke, D., und W. P. Rowe: Die Interferenz zwischen dem Polyoma-Virus und dem Stomatitis-vesicularis-Virus in der Maus. Arch. ges. Virusforsch. **15**, 210—219 (1965).

Feldman, H. A., and S. S. Wang: Sensitivity of various viruses to chloroform. Proc. Soc. exp. Biol. (N.Y.) **106**, 736—738 (1961).

Fenner, F.: In: The Biology of Animal Viruses, Vol. 1, p. 30. New York-London: Academic Press, 1968.

Field, E. J., and D. H. Adams: Riley virus in wild mice. Lancet **i**, 868 (1968).

Fitzmaurice, M. A., V. Riley, and G. A. Santisteban: Biological synergism between the LDH-virus and *Eperythrozoon coccoides*: studies on the mechanism. Path. et Biol. **20**, 743—750 (1972).

Fleisher, G. A., and K. G. Wakim: The fate of enzymes in body fluids — an experimental study. I. Disappearance rates of glutamic-pyruvic transaminase under various conditions. J. Lab. clin. Med. **61**, 76—85 (1963a).

Fleisher, G. A., and K. G. Wakim: Fate of enzymes in body fluids — an experimental study. III. Disappearance rates of glutamic-oxalacetic transaminase II under various conditions. J. Lab. clin. Med. **61**, 98—106 (1963b).

Franseen, C. C., and R. McLean: The phosphatase activity of tissues and plasma in tumors of bone. Amer. J. Cancer **24**, 299—317 (1941).

Frantsi, C., and K. F. Gregory: Reproduction of the lactate dehydrogenase-elevating (Riley) virus in mouse embryonic liver cell cultures. Virology **37**, 145—148 (1969).

FRIEND, C., and F. WRÓBLESKI: Lactic dehydrogenase activity of serum in mice with transplantable leukemia. Science **124**, 173—174 (1956).

GEORGII, A.: Die Aktivitätsänderung der Lactatdehydrogenase im Serum nach Infektion mit Geschwulstvirus der Maus als Regulationsstörung *in vivo*. Verh. dtsch. path. Ges. **46**, 357—358 (1962).

GEORGII, A.: Über das Lactatdehydrogenase-erhöhende Virus in Laboratoriumsgeschwülsten. Klin. Wschr. **42**, 559 —563 (1964).

GEORGII, A., H. BAYERLE, D. BRDICZKA und H. ZOBL: Über ein die Lactatdehydrogenase im Serum aktivierendes Virus aus Geschwülsten der Maus. Z. Krebsforsch. **65**, 334—341 (1963).

GEORGII, A., und D. BRDICZKA: Die Überlebenszeit des Lactatdehydrogenase-Agens aus Mäusegeschwülsten in Fibroblastenkulturen bei längerer Inkubation. Z. Krebsforsch. **66**, 207—212 (1964).

GEORGII, A., P. GOLDBRUNNER und D. BRDICZKA: Der Einfluß von p-Aminosalicylat bei der Nucleinsäureisolierung auf das Lactatdehydrogenase aktivierende Virus des Mäusetumors Serkon I. Naturwissenschaften **51**, 66 (1964).

GEORGII, A., M. JÄGER, H. KROTH und H. BAYERLE: Activitätsänderungen der Lactatdehydrogenase im Mäuseplasma durch Beimpfung mit virushaltigen Geschwulstfiltraten oder virushaltigen Gewebekulturen. Experientia (Basel) **18**, 71—72 (1962).

GEORGII, A., und I. KIRSCHENHOFER: Über die Isolierung von Lactat-Dehydrogenase-erhöhendem Virus aus wilden Mäusen. Z. Naturforsch. **20 b**, 1310 (1965).

GEORGII, A., H. KROTH und H. BAYERLE: Weitere Untersuchungen über die Aktivierung der Lactatdehydrogenase im Serum durch ein Geschwulstvirus der Maus. Klin. Wschr. **40**, 363 (1962).

GEORGII, A., and I. LENZ: Failure to propagate a lactic dehydrogenase-elevating agent from mice tumours in mice embryo cultures. Nature (Lond.) **202**, 1228—1229 (1964).

GEORGII, A., I. LENZ, and H. ZOBEL: Penetration of the placental barrier by the lactate dehydrogenase-elevating virus (Riley) and its behaviour in mouse embryo cultures following infection in utero. Proc. Soc. exp. Biol. (N.Y.) **117**, 322—326 (1964).

GEORGII, A. und L. THORN: Die Wirkung von Lactat-Dehydrogenase-erhöhendem Virus (Riley-Virus) bei Mäusen mit primären und transplantierten Carcinomen. Z. Krebsforsch. **67**, 156—165 (1965).

GEORGII, A., L. THORN und H. WRBA: Die Replikation von Riley's Enzym-erhöhendem Virus in embryonalen Mäusefibroblasten. Z. Naturforsch. **21 b**, 298 (1966a).

GEORGII, A., L. THORN, and H. WRBA: Action of Riley's enzyme-elevating virus on tumour-bearing mice. Nature (Lond.) **209**, 929—930 (1966b).

GEVAUDAN, P., R. GAY et G. ARNAUD: Étude sur l'activité de la transaminase glutamique-oxalacétique dans les cellules KB en culture normale et après inoculation avec un virus apparenté de la chorioméningite. Maroc méd. **435**, 1033—1041 (1961).

GEVAUDAN, P., G. GEVAUDAN, R. GAY et G. ARNAUD: Étude sur l'activité de la transaminase glutamique-oxalacétique dans les cellules KB en cultures normale et après inoculation de polio virus. Maroc méd. **418**, 219—229 (1960).

GIBBS, A. J.: Comparison of bee chronic paralysis virus with mouse lactic dehydrogenase virus. J. gen. Virol. **5**, 447—449 (1969).

GIBBS, A. J., B. D. HARRISON, D. H. WATSON, and P. WILDY: What's in a virus name? Nature (Lond.) **209**, 450—454 (1966).

GIERER, A., and G. SCHRAMM: Infectivity of ribonucleic acid from tobacco mosaic virus. Nature (Lond.) **177**, 702—703 (1956).

GILBERT, V. E.: Enzyme release from tissue cultures as an indicator of cellular injury by viruses. Virology **21**, 609—616 (1963).

GINOZA, W.: The effects of ionizing radiation on nucleic acids of bacteriophages and bacterial cells. Ann. Rev. Microbiol. **21**, 325—368 (1967).

GIUSTI, G., und F. PICCININO: Beobachtungen über die Plasma-Triosephosphat-Isomerase-Aktivität bei Lebererkrankungen. Acta hepato-splenol. (Stuttg.) **10**, 166—175 (1963).

GLEDHILL, A. W., D. L. J. BILBEY, and J. S. F. NIVEN: Effect of certain murine pathogens on phagocytic activity. Brit. J. exp. Path. **46**, 433—442 (1965).

112 References

GLEDHILL, A. W., and K. E. K. ROWSON: Unpublished data (1965).
GOTTSCHALK, R. G., H. H. GRANTHAM, and P. O. MILLER: Serum lactate dehydrogenase of chickens with sarcoma 13. Cancer Res. 25, 919—921 (1965).
GREEN, M.: Chemistry and structure of animal virus particles. Amer. J. Med. 38, 651 to 668 (1965).
GUTMAN, A. B.: Serum alkaline phosphatase activity in diseases of the skeletal and hepatobiliary systems. Amer. J. Med. 27, 875—901 (1959).
GUTMAN, A. B., and E. B. GUTMAN: An "acid" phosphatase occurring in the serum of patients with metastasizing carcinoma of the prostate gland. J. clin. Invest. 17, 473—478 (1938).
HALPERN, B. N., G. BIOZZI, T. NICOL, and D. L. J. BILBEY: Effect of experimental biliary obstruction on the phagocytic activity of the reticulo-endothelial system. Nature (Lond.) 180, 503—504 (1957).
HANNA, M. G., A. K. SZAKAL, and R. L. TYNDALL: Histoproliferative effect of Rauscher leukemia virus on lymphatic tissue: histological and ultrastructural studies of germinal centers and their relation to leukemogenesis. Cancer Res. 30, 1748—1763 (1970).
HANNA, M. G., H. E. WALBURG, R. L. TYNDALL, and M. J. SNODGRASS: Histoproliferative effect of Rauscher leukemia virus on lymphatic tissue. II. Antigen-stimulated germfree and conventional BALB/c mice. Proc. Soc. exp. Biol. (N.Y.) 134, 1132—1141 (1970).
HILL, B. R., and C. LEVI: Elevation of a serum component in neoplastic disease. Cancer Res. 14, 513—515 (1954).
HILL, B. R., and R. T. JORDAN: Serum lactic dehydrogenase activity in mice with transplantable leukemia. Cancer Res. 17, 144—147 (1957).
HILL, B. R., K. TANAKA, and E. ROBERTS: Elevation of plasma lactic dehydrogenase in mice receiving Moloney virus. Proc. Amer. Ass. Cancer Res. 3, 328 (1962).
HIRSCH, M. S., A. C. ALLISON, and J. J. HARVEY: Immune complexes in mice infected neonatally with Moloney leukaemogenic and murine sarcoma virus. Nature (Lond.) 223, 739—740 (1969).
HSIEH, K. M., V. SUNTZEFF, and E. V. COWDRY: Comparative study of serum lactic dehydrogenase activity in mice with transplanted and induced tumors. Cancer Res. 16, 237—239 (1956).
HORZINEK, M. C.: Comparative aspects of togaviruses. J. gen. Virol. 20, Supplement, pp. 87—103 (1973).
HORZINEK, M., and M. MUSSGAY: Studies on the nucleocapsid structure of a group A arbovirus. J. Virol. 4, 514—520 (1969).
HOWARD, R. J., A. L. NOTKINS, and S. E. MERGENHAGEN: Inhibition of cellular immune reactions in mice infected with lactic dehydrogenase virus. Nature (Lond.) 221, 873—874 (1969).
ISAACS, A.: Particle counts and infectivity titrations for animal viruses. Advanc.Virus Res. 4, 111—158 (1957).
JACOBSON, K. B., and K. NISHIO: Studies on plasma lactic dehydrogenase in mice with myeloid leukemia. II. On the site of production of the enzyme. Cancer Res. 23, 344—348 (1963).
KAMPSCHMIDT, R. F., H. F. UPCHURCH, and H. L. JOHNSON: Plasma enzymes in tumor-bearing rats. Cancer Res. 26, 237—240 (1966).
KARMEN, A., F. WRÓBLEWSKI, and J. S. LA DUE: Transaminase activity in human blood. J. clin. Invest 34, 126—133 (1955).
KEIR, H. M.: Virus-induced enzymes in mammalian cells infected with DNA-viruses. In: The Molecular Biology of Viruses, pp. 67—99, 18th Symp. Soc. gen. Microbiol. (L. V. CRAWFORD and M. P. G. STOKER, eds.). Cambridge Univ. Press, 1968.
KEKKI, M., and A. EISALO: Turnover of $^{35}$S-labelled serum albumin and gamma globulin in the rat: comparison of the resolution of plasma radioactivity curves by graphic means (manually) and by computer. Ann. Med. exp. Fenn. 42, 196—208 (1964).
KELLY, R., and D. GREIFF: The level of lactic dehydrogenase activity as an indicator of the growth of influenza virus in the embryonate egg. J. exp. Med. 113, 125—129 (1961).

KENNEDY, S. I. T., and D. C. BURKE: Studies on the structural proteins of Semliki Forest virus. J. gen. Virol. **14**, 87—98 (1972).

KING, E. J.: Introductory remarks to the symposium. Amer. J. Med. **27**, 849—860 (1959).

KING, E. J., and D. M. CAMPBELL: International enzyme units an attempt at international agreement. Clin. chim. Acta **6**, 301—306 (1961).

KING, E. J., and D. W. MOSS: International enzyme units and isoenzyme nomenclature. J. clin. Path. **16**, 391—393 (1963).

LATNER, A. L., P. S. GARDNER, D. M. TURNER, and J. O. BROWN: Effect of a possible oncogenic virus (adenovirus type 12) on lactate dehydrogenase in tissue culture. Lancet i, 197—198 (1964).

LEA, D. E.: Actions of Radiations on living Cells. London-New York: Cambridge Univ. Press, 1946.

LEADER, R. W., and A. I. HURVITZ: Interspecies patterns of slow virus diseases. Ann. Rev. Med. **23**, 191—200 (1972).

LEVY, H. B., D. AXELROD, and S. BARON: Messenger RNA for interferon production. Proc. Soc. exp. Biol. (N.Y.) **118**, 384—385 (1965).

LEVY, J. P., M. BOIRON, D. SILVESTRE, and J. BERNARD: The ultrastructure of Rauscher virus. Virology **26**, 146—150 (1965).

LURIA, S. E., R. C. WILLIAMS, and R. C. BACKUS: Electron micrographic counts of bacteriophage particles. J. Bact. **61**, 179—188 (1951).

MAEYER, E. DE, and J. DE MAEYER GUINGUARD: Contribution to U.I.C.C. Cancer Conference on "Cellular Control Mechanisms and Cancer". Amsterdam, 1963.

MAHY, B. W. J.: Unpublished data (1963).

MAHY, B. W. J.: Action of Riley's plasma enzyme-elevating virus in mice. Virology **24**, 481—483 (1964).

MAHY, B. W. J., J. J. HARVEY, and K. E. K. ROWSON: Some physical properties of a murine sarcoma virus (Harvey). Tex. Rep. Biol. Med. **24**, 620—628 (1966).

MAHY, B. W. J., C. W. PARR, and K. E. K. ROWSON: Increased plasma isomerase and transaminase activity in mice infected with lactic dehydrogenase-elevating virus. Nature (Lond.) **198**, 885 (1963a).

MAHY, B. W. J., C. W. PARR, and K. E. K. ROWSON: Plasma enzyme levels in mice infected with various viruses. J. gen. Microbiol. **32**, 1 (1963b).

MAHY, B. W. J., and K. E. K. ROWSON: Isoenzymic specificity of impaired clearance in mice infected with Riley virus. Science **149**, 756—757 (1965).

MAHY, B. W. J., K. E. K. ROWSON, and C. W. PARR: Effect of Riley's plasma enzyme-elevating virus (RV) on control of plasma enzyme levels in mice. Proc. biochem. Soc., Biochem. J. **95**, 19—20P (1965).

MAHY, B. W. J., K. E. K. ROWSON, and C. W. PARR: Studies on the mechanism of action of Riley virus. IV. The reticuloendothelial system and impaired plasma enzyme clearance in infected mice. J. exp. Med. **125**, 277—288 (1967).

MAHY, B. W. J., K. E. K. ROWSON, C. W. PARR, and M. H. SALAMAN: Studies on the mechanism of action of Riley virus. I. Action of substances effecting the reticulo-endothelial system on plasma enzyme levels in mice. J. exp. Med. **122**, 967—981 (1965).

MAHY, B. W. J., K. E. K. ROWSON, M. H. SALAMAN, and C. W. PARR: Plasma enzyme levels in virus infected mice. Virology **23**, 528—541 (1964).

MAHY, B. W. J., and E. D. WACHSMUTH: Studies on the clearance of lactic dehydrogenase (LDH) isoenzymes from plasma of normal mice and mice infected with lactic dehydrogenase virus (LDV). J. med. Microbiol. **6**, Px (1973).

MANSO, C., K. SUGIURA, and F. WRÓBLEWSKI: Glutathione reductase and lactic dehydrogenase activities of tissues of rodents with transplantable tumors. Cancer Res. **18**, 682—686 (1958).

MARCUS, P. I., and D. H. CARVER: Intrinsic interference: a new type of viral interference. J. Virol. **1**, 334—343 (1967).

MARCUS, P. I., and D. H. CARVER: Hemadsorption-negative plaque test for viruses inducing intrinsic interference. In: Fundamental Techniques in Virology, pp. 161—183 (K. HABEL and N. P. SALZMAN, eds.). New York-London: Academic Press, 1969.

MASSARRAT, S.: Enzyme kinetics, half-life, and immunological properties of iodine-131-labelled transaminases in pig blood. Nature (Lond.) **206**, 508—509 (1965).

MELNICK, J. L.: Classification and nomenclature of animal viruses. Progr. med. Virol. **13**, 462—484 (1971).

MERGENHAGEN, S. E., A. L. NOTKINS, and S. F. DOUGHERTY: Adjuvanticity of lactic dehydrogenase virus: influence of virus infection on the establishment of immunologic tolerance to a protein antigen in adult mice. J. Immunol. **99**, 576—581 (1967).

MERICAS, G., E. ANAGNOSTOU, ST. HADZIYANNIS, and S. KAKARI: The diagnostic value of serum leucine aminopeptidase. J. clin. Path. **17**, 52—55 (1964).

MICHAELIDES, M. C., and S. SCHLESINGER: Structural proteins of lactic dehydrogenase virus. Virology **55**, 211—217 (1973).

MICHAELIDES, M. C., and S. SCHLESINGER: Effect of acute or chronic infection with lactic dehydrogenase virus (LDV) on the susceptibility of mice to plasmacytoma MOPC-315. J. Immunol. **112**, 1560—1564 (1974).

MIMS, C. A.: Aspects of the pathogenesis of virus diseases. Bact. Rev. **28**, 30—71 (1964).

MUNDY, J., and P. C. WILLIAMS: Transmissible agent associated with some mouse neoplasms. Science **134**, 834—835 (1961).

NICOL, T., D. L. J. BILBEY, J. CORDINGLEY, and C. DRUCE: Response of the reticulo-endothelial system to stimulation with oestrogens. Nature (Lond.) **192**, 978—979 (1961).

NICOL, T., and D. L. J. BILBEY: Reversal by diethyl-stilboestrol of the depressant effect of cortisone on the phagocytic activity of the reticulo-endothelial system. Nature (Lond.) **179**, 1137—1138 (1957).

NIWA, A., S. YAMAZAKI, J. BADER, and A. L. NOTKINS: Incorporation of labelled precursors into RNA and protein of lactic dehydrogenase virus. J. Virol. **12**, 401—404 (1973).

NOTKINS, A. L.: Studies on the properties and transmission of the lactic dehydrogenase agent. Proc. Amer. Ass. Cancer Res. **4**, 48 (1963a).

NOTKINS, A. L.: Relationship between the multiplication of lactic dehydrogenase agent and plasma enzyme activity. Fed. Proc. **22**, 487 (1963b).

NOTKINS, A. L.: Recovery of an infectious ribonucleic acid from the lactic dehydrogenase agent by treatment with ether. Virology **22**, 563—567 (1964a).

NOTKINS, A. L.: Recovery of an infectious nucleic acid from the lactic dehydrogenase agent by extraction with ether, chloroform or butanol. Fed. Proc. **23**, 131 (1964b).

NOTKINS, A. L.: Lactic dehydrogenase virus. Bact. Rev. **29**, 143—160 (1965a).

NOTKINS, A. L.: Studies on the mechanism of enzyme elevation in mice infected with the lactic dehydrogenase virus. Fed. Proc. **24**, 378 (1965b).

NOTKINS, A. L.: Recovery of an infectious ribonucleic acid from the lactic dehydrogenase virus following extraction with butanol or chloroform. Biochim. biophys. Acta (Amst.) **103**, 509—511 (1965c).

NOTKINS, A. L.: Infectious virus-antibody complexes during chronic viremia. Proc. 9th Int. Cancer Congr., Tokyo, p. 310 (1966a).

NOTKINS, A. L.: Catabolism of γ-globulin and increased antibody production in mice infected with lactic dehydrogenase virus. Proc. 9th Int. Congr. Microbiol., p. 628, Moscow, 1966b.

NOTKINS, A. L.: Infectious virus-antibody complex. Fed. Proc. **25**, 615 (1966c).

NOTKINS, A. L.: Neutralization of sensitized virus by anti-gammaglobulin. Perspect. Virol. **6**, 189—192 (1968).

NOTKINS, A. L.: Enzymatic and immunologic alterations in mice infected with lactic dehydrogenase virus. Amer. J. Path. **64**, 733—746 (1971a).

NOTKINS, A. L.: Infectious virus-antibody complexes-interaction with anti-immunoglobulins, complement, and rheumatoid factor. J. exp. Med. **134**, 41s—51s (1971b).

NOTKINS, A. L., R. J. BERRY, J. B. MOLONEY, and R. E. GREENFIELD: Relationship of the lactic dehydrogenase factor to certain murine tumors. Nature (Lond.) **193**, 79—80 (1962).

NOTKINS, A. L., and M. COSMIDES: The effect of heparin on the titer of the infectious nucleic acid from the lactic dehydrogenase agent. Biochim. biophys. Acta (Amst.) **91**, 536—538 (1964).

NOTKINS, A. L., and R. E. GREENFIELD: Infection of tumor-bearing mice with the lactic dehydrogenase agent. Proc. Soc. exp. Biol. (N.Y.) **109**, 988—991 (1962a).

NOTKINS, A. L., and R. E. GREENFIELD: The lactic dehydrogenase factor in the tumor-bearing animal. Proc. Amer. Ass. Cancer Res. **3**, 348 (1962b).

NOTKINS, A. L., R. E. GREENFIELD, D. MARSHALL, and L. BANE: Multiple enzyme changes in the plasma of normal and tumor-bearing mice following infection with the lactic dehydrogenase agent. J. exp. Med. **117**, 185—195 (1963).

NOTKINS, A. L., M. MAGE, W. K. ASHE, and S. MAHAR: Neutralization of sensitized lactic dehydrogenase virus by anti-γ-globulin. J. Immunol. **100**, 314—320 (1968).

NOTKINS, A. L., S. MAHAR, C. SCHEELE, and J. GOFFMAN: Infectious virus-antibody complex in the blood of chronically infected mice. J. exp. Med. **124**, 81—97 (1966).

NOTKINS, A. L., S. E. MERGENHAGEN, and R. J. HOWARD: Effect of virus infections on the function of the immune system. Ann. Rev. Microbiol. **24**, 525—538 (1970).

NOTKINS, A. L., S. E. MERGENHAGEN, A. A. RIZZO, C. SCHEELE, and T. A. WALDMANN: Elevated γ-globulin and increased antibody production in mice infected with lactic dehydrogenase virus. J. exp. Med. **123**, 347—364 (1966).

NOTKINS, A. L., and C. SCHEELE: An infectious nucleic acid from the lactic dehydrogenase agent. Virology **20**, 640—642 (1963a).

NOTKINS, A. L., and C. SCHEELE: Studies on the transmission and the excretion of the lactic dehydrogenase agent. J. exp. Med. **118**, 7—12 (1963b).

NOTKINS, A. L., and C. SCHEELE: Impaired clearance of enzymes in mice infected with the lactic dehydrogenase agent. J. nat. Cancer Inst. **33**, 741—749 (1964).

NOTKINS, A. L., C. SCHEELE, and H. W. SCHERP: Transmission of the lactic dehydrogenase agent in normal and partially edentulous mice. Nature (Lond.) **202**, 418—419 (1964).

NOTKINS, A. L., and S. J. SHOCHAT: Studies on the multiplication and the properties of the lactic dehydrogenase agent. J. exp. Med. **117**, 735—747 (1963).

OLD, L. J., B. BENACERRAF, D. A. CLARKE, E. A. CARSWELL, and E. STOCKERT: The role of the reticuloendothelial system in the host reaction to neoplasia. Cancer Res. **21**, 1281—1301 (1961).

OLD, L. J., C. IRITANI, E. STOCKERT, E. A. BOYSE, and H. A. CAMPBELL: Increased antileukemic activity of E. coli asparaginase in mice infected with L.D.H.-elevating virus. Lancet **ii**, 684—685 (1968).

OLDSTONE, M. B. A., and F. J. DIXON: Pathogenesis of chronic disease associated with persistant lymphocytic choriomeningitis viral infection. J. exp. Med. **129**, 483—505 (1969).

OLDSTONE, M. B. A., and F. J. DIXON: Inhibition of antibodies to nuclear antigen and to DNA in New Zealand mice infected with lactate dehydrogenase virus. Science **175**, 784—786 (1972).

OLDSTONE, M. B. A., and F. J. DIXON: Lactic dehydrogenase virus-induced immune complex type of glomerulonephritis. J. Immunol. **106**, 1260—1263 (1971).

OLDSTONE, M. B. A., A. TISHON, and J. M. CHILLER: Chronic virus infection and immune responsiveness. II. Lactic dehydrogenase virus infection and immune response to non-viral antigens. J. Immunol. **112**, 370—375 (1974).

OLDSTONE, M. B. A., S. YAMAZAKI, A. NIWA, and A. L. NOTKINS: *In vitro* detection of cells infected with lactic dehydrogenase virus (LDV) by fluorescein-labelled antibody to LDV. Intervirology **2**, 261—265 (1974).

PHILLIPS, A., and J. BOYD: Blood clearance of asparaginase and tumor inhibition in mice infected with the lactic dehydrogenase-elevating virus. Bact. Proc., p. 153 (1969).

PLAGEMANN, P. G. W., K. F. GREGORY, H. E. SWIM, and K. K. W. CHAN: Plasma lactic dehydrogenase-elevating agent of mice: distribution in tissues and effect on lactic dehydrogenase isozyme patterns. Canad. J. Microbiol. **9**, 75—86 (1963).

PLAGEMANN, P. G. W., and H. E. SWIM: Studies of virus associated with metabolic disease in mice. Proc. 8th Int. Congr. Microbiol., p. 91, Montreal, 1962.

PLAGEMANN, P. G. W., and H. E. SWIM: Studies of the plasma lactic dehydrogenase-elevating virus (PLDEV) of mice. Proc. Amer. Ass. Cancer Res. **4**, 53 (1963).

PLAGEMANN, P. G. W., and H. E. SWIM: Propagation of lactic dehydrogenase-elevating virus in cell culture. Proc. Soc. exp. Biol. (N.Y.) **121**, 1147—1152 (1966a).

PLAGEMANN, P. G. W., and H. E. SWIM: Relationship between the lactic dehydrogenase-elevating virus and transplantable murine tumors. Proc. Soc. exp. Biol. (N.Y.) **121**, 1142—1146 (1966b).

PLAGEMANN, P. G. W., M. WATANABE, and H. E. SWIM: Plasma lactic dehydrogenase-elevating agent of mice: effect on levels of additional enzymes. Proc. Soc. exp. Biol. (N.Y.) **111**, 749—754 (1962).

POLSON, A., and M. H. V. VAN REGENMORTEL: A new method for determination of sedimentation constants of viruses. Virology **15**, 397—403 (1961).

POPE, J. H.: Studies of a virus isolated from a wild house mouse, *mus musculus*, and producing splenomegaly and lymph node enlargement in mice. Aust. J. exp. Biol. med. Sci. **39**, 521—536 (1961).

POPE, J. H.: Detection of an avirulent virus apparently related to Friend virus. Aust. J. exp. Biol. med. Sci. **41**, 349—362 (1963).

POPE, J. H., and W. P. ROWE: Identification of WMI as LDH virus, and its recovery from wild mice in Maryland. Proc. Soc. exp. Biol. (N.Y.) **116**, 1015—1019 (1964).

PORTER, D. D.: Quantitative view of the slow virus landscape. Progr. med. Virol. **13**, 339—372 (1971).

PORTER, D. D., and H. G. PORTER: Deposition of immune complexes in the kidneys of mice infected with lactic dehydrogenase virus. J. Immunol. **106**, 1264—126 (1971).

PORTER, D. D., H. G. PORTER, and B. B. DEERHAKE: Immunofluorescence assay for antigen and antibody in lactic dehydrogenase virus infection of mice. J. Immunol. **102**, 431—436 (1969).

PROFFITT, M. R., and C. C. CONGDON: The effect of a large dose of LDH virus on mouse lymphatic tissue. Fed. Proc. **29**, 559 (1970).

PROFFITT, M. R., C. C. CONGDON, and R. L. TYNDALL: The combined action of Rauscher leukemia virus and lactic dehydrogenase virus on mouse lymphatic tissue. Int. J. Cancer **9**, 193—211 (1972).

PROSSER, P. R., and R. EVANS: An electron microscopic study of lactic dehydrogenase virus in cultures of mouse peritoneal macrophages. J. gen. Virol. **1**, 419—424 (1967).

RAUEN, H. M. und H. HUPE: Das Lactatdehydrogenase-Agens im Blute tumortragender Mäuse. Arzneimittel-Forsch. **13**, 933—936 (1963).

REICHARD, H.: Ornithine carbamyl transferase activity in human serum in diseases of the liver and the biliary system. J. Lab. clin. Med. **57**, 78—87 (1961).

RICHTER, A., and E. WECKER: The reaction of EEE virus preparations with sodium deoxycholate. Virology **20**, 263—268 (1963).

RILEY, V.: Adaptation of orbital bleeding technic to rapid serial blood studies. Proc. Soc. exp. Biol. (N.Y.) **104**, 751—754 (1960).

RILEY, V.: Virus-tumor synergism. Science **134**, 666—668 (1961).

RILEY, V.: Synergistic glycolytic activity associated with transmissible agents and neoplastic growth. J. gen. Physiol. **45**, 614A—615A (1962a).

RILEY, V.: Role of viruses in glycolysis of tumors and hosts. Fed. Proc., pp. 21—87 (1962b).

RILEY, V.: Evidence for a minute infectious entity. Proc. Amer. Ass. Cancer Res. **4**, 57 (1963a).

RILEY, V.: Enzymatic determination of transmissible replicating factors associated with mouse tumors. Ann. N.Y. Acad. Sci. **100**, 762—789 (1963b).

RILEY, V.: Transmissible agents and anaemia of mouse cancer. N.Y. State J. Med. **63**, 1523—1531 (1963c).

RILEY, V.: Synergistic glycolytic activity associated with transmissible agents and neoplastic growth. In: Control Mechanisms in Respiration and Fermentation, pp. 211—241 (BARBARA WRIGHT, ed.). New York: Ronald Press, 1963d.

RILEY, V.: Synergism between a lactate dehydrogenase-elevating virus and *Eperythrozoon coccoides*. Science **146**, 921—923 (1964).

RILEY, V.: Discussion following a paper by Pollard, M., on "Neoplasia in germ-free animals". Perspect. Virol. **4**, 265 (1965).

RILEY, V.: Spontaneous mammary tumors: decrease of incidence in mice infected with an enzyme-elevating virus. Science **153**, 1657—1658 (1966a).

RILEY, V.: Le virus elevant le taux de la deshydrogenase lactique. Thesis monograph University of Paris (1966b).

RILEY, V.: Role of the LDH-elevating virus in leukemia therapy by asparaginase. Nature (Lond.) **220**, 1245—1246 (1968a).

RILEY, V.: Lactate dehydrogenase in the normal and malignant state in mice and the influence of a benign enzyme-elevating virus. In: Methods in Cancer Research (HARRIS BUSCH, ed.) **4**, 493—618, 1968b, Academic Press.

RILEY, V.: Asparaginase therapy: influence of the LDH-virus. Proc. Amer. Ass. Cancer Res. **10**, 73 (1969).

RILEY, V.: Influence of a benign virus upon mouse leukemia during asparaginase therapy. Path. et Biol. **18**, 757—764 (1970).

RILEY, V.: Rescue of an eclipsed LDH-virus by host immunosuppression techniques. Fed. Proc. **30**, 1100 (1971).

RILEY, V.: Persistence and other characteristics of the lactate-dehydrogenase-elevating virus (LDH-virus). Progr. med. Virol. **18**, 198—213 (1974a).

RILEY, V.: Biological contaminants and scientific misinterpretations (viruses). Cancer Res. **34**, 1752—1754 (1974b).

RILEY, V.: Erroneous interpretation of valid experimental observations through interference by the LDH virus. J. nat. Cancer Inst. **52**, 1673—1677 (1974c).

RILEY, V., H. A. CAMPBELL, J. D. LOVELESS, and M. A. FITZMAURICE: Density gradient centrifugation and molecular sieve studies of lactic dehydrogenase-elevating virus-like agent. Proc. Amer. Ass. Cancer Res. **5**, 53 (1964).

RILEY, V., H. A. CAMPBELL, and C. C. STOCK: Asparaginase clearance: influence of the LDH-elevating virus. Proc. Soc. exp. Biol. (N.Y.) **133**, 38—42 (1970).

RILEY, V. and M. A. FITZMAURICE: "Helper" influence of the LDH-virus in the production of leukaemia by attenuated Rauscher virus. Proc. Amer. Ass. Cancer Res. **14**, 112 (1973).

RILEY, V., M. A. FITZMAURICE, J. D. LOVELESS, T. G. KRYZAK, M. R. GALLAGHER, and W. M. SILER: Mechanism of plasma enzyme elevation observed with virus infection and neoplastic growth. Proc. Amer. Ass. Cancer Res. **6**, 54 (1965).

RILEY, V., E. HUERTO, D. BARDELL, M. A. FITZMAURICE, and J. D. LOVELESS: Studies on the origin of elevated plasma lactic dehydrogenase (LDH). Fed. Proc. **22**, 242 (1963).

RILEY, V., E. HUERTO, D. BARDELL, J. D. LOVELESS, and M. A. FITZMAURICE: Influence of LDH-elevating virus on normal and tumor-bearing hosts. Proc. Amer. Ass. Cancer Res. **3**, 354 (1962).

RILEY, V., E. HUERTO, J. D. LOVELESS, D. BARDELL, M. FITZMAURICE, and C. FORMAN: Inapparent transmissible agents in oncology and their influence on tumor and host. Acta Un. int. Cancr. **19**, 263—270 (1963).

RILEY, V., E. HUERTO, F. LILLY, D. BARDELL, J. D. LOVELESS, and M. A. FITZMAURICE: Some characteristics of virus-like entities associated with 30 varieties of experimental tumor. Proc. Amer. Ass. Cancer Res. **3**, 262 (1961).

RILEY, V., F. LILLY, E. HUERTO, and D. BARDELL: Transmissible agent associated with 26 types of experimental mouse neoplasms. Science **132**, 545—547 (1960).

RILEY, V., J. D. LOVELESS, and M. A. FITZMAURICE: Comparison of a lactate dehydrogenase elevating virus-like agent and *Eperythrozoon coccoides*. Proc. Soc. exp. Biol. (N.Y.) **116**, 486—490 (1964).

RILEY, V., J. D. LOVELESS, M. A. FITZMAURICE, and W. M. SILER: Mechanism of lactate dehydrogenase (LDH) elevation in virus infected hosts. Life Sci. **4**, 487—507 (1965).

RILEY, V., J. D. LOVELESS, M. A. FITZMAURICE, I. SMULLYAN, and S. W. FISCHER: Characteristics of the Friend's leukemia disease in the presence and absence of a benign enzyme-elevating (LDH) virus. Proc. Amer. Ass. Cancer Res. **8**, 56 (1967).

RILEY, V. and D. SPECKMAN: Influence of the LDH-virus on the neoplastic process. XI Int. Cancer Congr. Abst. p. 676 (1974).

RILEY, V., D. H. SPECKMAN, and M. A. FITZMAURICE: Influence of asparaginase and glutaminase upon free amino acids in normal and tumor-bearing mice. Colloques Internationaux C.N.R.S., No. 197, pp. 139—158 (1970a).

RILEY, V., D. H. SPECKMAN, and M. A. FITZMAURICE: Critical influence of an enzyme-elevating virus upon long-term remissions of mouse leukemia following asparaginase therapy. Recent Results in Cancer Res. 33, 81—101 (1970b).

RILEY, V., D. H. SPECKMAN, M. A. FITZMAURICE: Influence of the LDH-elevating virus in revealing profound alterations in host physiology during asparaginase therapy. Proc. Amer. Ass. Cancer Res. 12, 64 (1971).

RILEY, V., D. H. SPECKMAN, M. A. FITZMAURICE, J. ROBERTS, J. S. HOLCENBERG, and W. C. DOLOWY: Studies on a new glutaminase/asparaginase: therapeutic properties, half life, and alterations in the plasma amino acids. Proc. Amer. Ass. Cancer Res. 13, 117 (1972).

RILEY, V., D. H. SPECKMAN, M. A. FITZMAURICE, J. ROBERTS, J. S. HOLCENBERG, and W. C. DOLOWY: Therapeutic properties of a new glutaminase-asparaginase preparation and the influence of the lactate dehydrogenase-elevating virus. Cancer Res. 34, 429—438 (1974).

RILEY, V., D. H. SPECKMAN, M. A. FITZMAURICE, and C. N. LULHAM: Possible mechanism for permanent remissions of leukemia in mice treated with L-asparaginase. Xth Int. Cancer Congr. Proc., pp. 445—446 (1970).

RILEY, V., and F. WRÓBLEWSKI: Serial lactic dehydrogenase activity in plasma of mice with growing or regressing tumors. Science 132, 151—152 (1960).

ROBERTS, W. M.: Variations of the phosphatase activity of the blood in disease. Brit. J. exp. Path. 11, 90—95 (1930).

ROBERTS, W. M.: Blood phosphatase and the van den Bergh reaction in the differentiation of the several types of jaundice. Brit. Med. J. i, 734—738 (1933).

ROE, F. J. C., and K. E. K. ROWSON: The induction of cancer by combinations of viruses and other agents. Int. Rev. exp. Path. 6, 181—227 (1968).

ROSE, A., M. WEST, and H. J. ZIMMERMAN: Serum enzymes in disease. V. Isocitric dehydrogenase, malic dehydrogenase and glycolytic enzymes in patients with carcinoma of the breast. Cancer 14, 726—733 (1961).

ROWE, W. P.: Resistance of mice infected with Moloney leukemia virus to Friend virus infection. Science 141, 40—41 (1963).

ROWE, W. P., J. W. HARTLEY, and R. J. HUEBNER: Polyoma and other indigenous mouse viruses. In: The Problems of Laboratory Animal Diseases (R. J. C. HARRIS, ed.), pp. 131—142. London-New York: Academic Press, 1962.

ROWE, W. P., F. A. MURPHY, G. H. BERGOLD, J. CASALS, J. HOTCHIN, K. M. JOHNSON, F. LEHMANN-GRUBE, C. A. MIMS, E. TRAUB, and P. A. WEBB: Arenoviruses: proposed name for a newly defined virus group. J. Virol. 5, 651—652 (1970).

ROWSON, K. E. K.: Transmission of RV from parents to offspring. Brit. Emp. Cancer Campaign Ann. Rep. 40, 205—206 (1962).

ROWSON, K. E. K.: Riley virus in wild mice, effect of drugs on replication of Riley viruses. Brit. Emp. Cancer Campaign Ann. Rep. 41, 222—223 (1963).

ROWSON, K. E. K.: Unpublished data (1964).

ROWSON, K. E. K.: Host range of RV. Brit. Emp. Cancer Campaign Ann. Rep. 44, 113 (1966).

ROWSON, K. E. K.: Decreased viraemia following injection of statalon. International Virology 1, 128, Basel: S. Karger, 1969.

ROWSON, K. E. K., D. H. ADAMS, and M. H. SALAMAN: Riley's enzyme-elevating virus; a study of the infection in mice and its relation to virus-induced leukemia. Acta Un. int. Cancr. 19, 404—406 (1963).

ROWSON, K. E. K., and R. W. HORNE: Unpublished data (1962).

ROWSON, K. E. K., and L. MICHAELS: Lactic dehydrogenase (LDH) virus and its localisation by immunofluorescence. J. med. Microbiol. 6, Pxi (1973).

ROWSON, K. E. K., and B. W. J. MAHY: The interaction between Riley's plasma enzyme elevating virus and the reticuloendothelial system. J. gen. Microbiol. 39, xi (1965).

Rowson, K. E. K., B. W. J. Mahy, and M. Bendinelli: Riley virus neutralizing activity in the plasma of infected mice with persistent viraemia. Virology **28**, 775 —778 (1966).

Rowson, K. E. K., B. W. J. Mahy, and R. Evans: Site of Riley virus replication, and the source of the excess plasma enzymes in infected mice. Brit. Emp. Cancer Campaign Ann. Rep. **41**, 227 (1963).

Rowson, K. E. K., B. W. J. Mahy, and M. H. Salaman: Size estimation by filtration of the enzyme-elevating virus of Riley. Life Sci. **2**, 479—485 (1963).

Rowson, K. E. K., B. W. J. Mahy, and M. H. Salaman: Studies on the mechanism of action of Riley virus. II. Action of substances affecting the reticuloendothelial system on the level of viraemia. J. exp. Med. **122**, 983—992 (1965).

Rowson, K. E. K., L. Michaels, and G. A. Hurst: Early changes in the kidneys of BALB/c mice infected with lactic dehydrogenase virus. Nature (Lond.) **248**, 686 to 687 (1974).

Rowson, K. E. K., I. B. Parr, and T. Alper: The radiation target size of Riley virus infectivity. J. gen. Microbiol. **50**, v (1968a).

Rowson, K. E. K., I. B. Parr, and T. Alper: Radiation target size of Riley virus. Virology **36**, 157—159 (1968b).

Rutenburg, A. M., J. A. Goldbarg, and E. P. Pineda: Serum γ-glutamyl transpeptidase activity in hepatobiliary pancreatic disease. Gastroenterology **45**, 43—48 (1963).

Salaman, M. H.: Immunodepression by viruses. Antibot. et Chemother. **15**, 393—406 (1969).

Salaman, M. H.: Immunodepression by mammalian viruses and plasmodia. Proc. roy. Soc. Med. **63**, 11—15 (1970).

Salaman, M. H., and N. Wedderburn: The immunodepressive effect of Friend virus. Immunology **10**, 445—458 (1966).

Salem, H., M. H. Grossman, and D. L. J. Bilbey: Micro-method for intravenous injection and blood sampling. J. pharm. Sci. **52**, 794—795 (1963).

Salthe, S. N., O. P. Chilson, and N. O. Kaplan: Hybridization of lactic dehydrogenase *in vivo* and *in vitro*. Nature (Lond.) **207**, 723—726 (1965).

Santisteban, G. A., V. Riley, and M. A. Fitzmaurice: Thymolytic and adrenal cortical responses to the LDH-elevating virus. Proc. Soc. exp. Biol. (N.Y.) **139**, 202—206 (1972).

Santisteban, G. A., V. Riley, and K. Willhight: Studies in virus-tumor relationships: responses of the adrenocortical-thymolymphatic system to the LDH-elevating virus. Abstracts, Tenth Int. Cancer Congr., p. 302. Medical Arts Publishing Co., Austin, 1970.

Schaffer, F. L.: Physical and chemical properties and infectivity of RNA from animal viruses. Cold Spr. Harb. Symp. quant. Biol. **27**, 89—99 (1962).

Schapira, F.; J.-C. Dreyfus et G. Schapira: La durée de séjour dans le plasma de l'aldolase chez le lapin: étude à l'aide d'une aldolase marquée à l'iode radioactif. Rev. franç. Études clin. biol. **7**, 829—832 (1962).

Schwartz, M. A., M. West, W. S. Walsh, and H. J. Zimmerman: Serum enzymes in disease. VIII. Glycolytic and oxidative enzymes and transaminases in patients with gastrointestinal carcinoma. Cancer **15**, 346—353 (1962).

Sibley, J. A., and A. L. Lehninger: Aldolase in the serum and tissues of tumor-bearing animals. J. nat. Cancer Inst. **9**, 303—309 (1949a).

Sibley, J. A., and A. L. Lehninger: Determination of aldolase in animal tissues. J. biol. Chem. **177**, 859—872 (1949b).

Snodgrass, M. J., and M. G. Hanna: Histoproliferative effect of Rauscher leukemia virus on lymphatic tissue. III. Alterations in the thymic-dependent area induced by the passenger lactic dehydrogenase virus. J. nat. Cancer Inst. **45**, 741—759 (1970).

Snodgrass, M. J., D. S. Lowrey, and M. G. Hanna: Changes induced by lactic dehydrogenase virus in thymus and thymus-dependent areas of lymphatic tissue. J. Immunol. **108**, 877—892 (1972).

SNODGRASS, M. J., J. M. YUHAS, and M. G. HANNA: Histoproliferative effect of Rauscher leukemia virus on lymphatic tissues. IV. Lactic dehydrogenase virus and erythropoietin potentiation of the erythroid response. J. nat. Cancer Inst. 50, 735—743 (1973).

SPECKMAN, D., and V. RILEY: E-N-Monomethyllysine and other plasma amino acids in leukemic mice and effects of asparaginase. Fed. Proc. 30, 1067 (1971).

SPECKMAN, D., and V. RILEY: Studies in leukemia: the levels of asparagine, glutamine, asparaginase and glutaminase in the mouse following asparaginase administration. Proc. Amer. Ass. Cancer Res. 13, 81 (1972).

SPECKMAN, D., V. RILEY, G. A. SANTISTEBAN, W. KIRK, and L. BREDBERG: The role of stress in producing elevated corticosterone levels and thymus involution in mice. XI Int. Cancer Congr. Abst., p. 382 (1974).

SPECKMAN, D. H., V. RILEY, and L. TESCHNER: Asparaginase therapy in leukemic mice: changes in plasma amino acids as modified by the LDH virus. Abstracts, Tenth Int. Cancer Congr., pp. 443—444 (1970).

SPIRIN, A. S.: Some problems concerning the macromolecular structure of ribonucleic acids. Progr. Nucl. Acid Res. 1, 301—345 (1963).

STANSLY, P. G.: Non-oncogenic infectious agents associated with experimental tumors. Progr. exp. Tumor Res. 7, 224—258 (1965).

STANSLY, P. G., and C. F. NEILSON: Relationship between spleen weight increase factor (SWIF) of mice and *Eperythrozoon coccoides*. Proc. Soc. exp. Biol. (N.Y.) 119, 1059—1063 (1965).

STARK, D. M., and C. G. CRISPENS: Studies on the multiplication of lactic dehydrogenase-elevating agents. Experientia (Basel) 21, 270 (1965).

STEEVES, R. A., E. A. MIRAND, S. THOMSON, and L. AVILA: Enhancement of spleen focus formation and virus replication in Friend virus infected mice. Cancer Res. 29, 1111—1116 (1969).

STUART, A. E.: The Reticulo-endothelial System. Edinburgh-London: E & S Livingstone, 1970.

TENNANT, R. W.: Taxonomy of murine viruses. Nat. Cancer Inst. Monograph No. 20, 47—53 (1966).

TENNANT, R. W., and T. G. WARD: Pneumonia virus of mice (PVM) in cell culture. Proc. Soc. exp. Biol. (N.Y.) 111, 395—398 (1962).

THOMPSON, W. R.: Use of moving averages and interpolation to estimate median-effective dose. 1. Fundamental formulas, estimation of error, and relation to other methods. Bact. Rev. 11, 115—145 (1947).

TURNER, W., P. S. EBERT, R. BASSIN, G. SPAHN, and M. A. CHIRIGOS: Potentiation of murine sarcoma virus (Harvey) (Moloney) oncogenicity in lactic dehydrogenase-elevating virus-infected mice. Proc. Soc. exp. Biol. (N.Y.) 136, 1314—1318 (1970).

UNANUE, E. R.: The regulatory role of macrophages in antigenic stimulation. Advanc. Immunol. 15, 95—165 (1972).

VAN DER HELM, H. J., H. A. ZONDAG, H. A. PH. HARTOG, and M. W. VAN DER KOOI: Lactic dehydrogenase isoenzymes in myocardial infarction. Clin. chim. Acta 7, 540 —544 (1962).

WACHSMUTH, E. D., and D. KLINGMUELLER: Immune response to lactate dehydrogenase (LDH) isoenzymes in normal mice and in mice infected with lactic dehydrogenase virus (LDV). J. med. Microbiol. 6, Px—Pxi (1973).

WACKER, W. E. C., and G. A. SCHOENENBERGER: Peptide inhibitors of lactic dehydrogenase (LDH) I: specific inhibition of LDH-$M_4$ and LDH-$H_4$ by inhibitor peptides I and II. Biochem. biophys. Res. Commun. 22, 291—296 (1966).

WAKIM, K. G., and G. A. FLEISHER: The fate of enzymes in body fluids — an experimental study. II. Disappearance rates of glutamic-oxalacetic transaminase I under various conditions. J. Lab. clin. Med. 61, 86—97 (1963a).

WAKIM, K. G., and G. A. FLEISHER: The fate of enzymes in body fluids — an experimental study. IV. Relationship of the reticuloendothelial system to activities and disappearance rates of various enzymes. J. Lab. clin. Med. 61, 107—119 (1973b).

WALLIS, C., and J. L. MELNICK: Thermal inactivation of poliovirus under anaerobic conditions. J. Bact. **84**, 389—392 (1962).

WARNOCK, M. L.: Isozymic patterns in organs of mice infected with LDH agent. Proc. Soc. exp. Biol. (N.Y.) **115**, 448—452 (1964).

WENNER, C. E., S. J. MILLIAN, E. A. MIRAND, and J. T. GRACE: Serum lactic dehydrogenase levels of mice inoculated with oncogenic and non-oncogenic viruses. Virology **18**, 486—487 (1962).

WESTAWAY, E. G.: Protein specified by group B togaviruses in mammalian cells during productive infections. Virology **51**, 454—465 (1973).

WILDY, P.: Classification and nomenclature of viruses. Monographs in Virology **5**, 1—81. Basel: S. Karger, 1971.

WILKINSON, J.H.: An Introduction to Diagnostic Enzymology. London: Edward Arnold, 1962.

WILNER, B. I.: A classification of the major groups of human and other animal viruses, 4th Ed. Minneapolis: Burgess Publishing Co., 1969.

WILSON, A. C., N. O. KAPLAN, L. LEVINE, A. PESCE, M. REICHLIN, and W. S. ALLISON: Evolution of lactic dehydrogenase. Fed. Proc. **23**, 1258—1266 (1964).

WOLFSON, S. K., J. A. SPENCER, R. L. STERKEL, and H. G. WILLIAMS-ASHMAN: Clinical and experimental studies on serum pyridine nucleotide-linked dehydrogenases in liver damages. Ann. N.Y. Acad. Sci. **75**, 260—269 (1958).

WRÓBLEWSKI, F.: The mechanisms of alteration in lactic dehydrogenase activity of body fluids. Ann. N.Y. Acad. Sci. **75**, 322—338 (1958).

WRÓBLEWSKI, F.: The significance of alterations in lactic dehydrogenase activity in body fluids in the diagnosis of malignant tumors. Cancer **12**, 27—39 (1959).

WRÓBLEWSKI, F., G. JERVIS, and J. S. LA DUE: The diagnostic, prognostic and epidemiologic significance of serum glutamic oxaloacetic transaminase (SGO-T) alterations in acute hepatitis. Ann. intern. Med. **45**, 782—800 (1956).

WRÓBLEWSKI, F., and J. S. LA DUE: Lactic dehydrogenase activity in blood. Proc. Soc. exp. Biol. (N.Y.) **90**, 210—213 (1955).

WRÓBLEWSKI, F., and J. S. LA DUE: Serum glutamic pyruvic transaminase (SGP-T) in hepatic disease: a preliminary report. Ann. intern. Med. **45**, 801—811 (1956).

YAFFE, D.: The distribution and *in vitro* propagation of an agent causing high plasma lactic dehydrogenase activity. Cancer Res. **22**, 573—580 (1962a).

YAFFE, D.: Studies on an agent associated with high plasma lactic dehydrogenase activity. Acta Un. int. Cancr. **19**, 407—409 (1962b).

YAMAZAKI, S., and A. L. NOTKINS: Inhibition of replication of lactic dehydrogenase virus by actinomycin. J. Virol. **11**, 473—478 (1973).

ZEBOVITZ, E., J. K. L. LEONG, and S. C. DOUGHTY: Japanese encephalitis virus replication: a procedure for the selective isolation and characterization of viral RNA species. Arch. ges. Virusforsch. **38**, 319—327 (1972).

ZEIGEL, R. F., and F. J. RAUSCHER: Electron microscopic and bioassay studies on a murine leukemia virus (Rauscher): preliminary report. J. nat. Cancer Inst. **30**, 207—219 (1963).

ZIMMERMAN, H. J., M. WEST, and P. HELLER: Serum enzymes in disease. II. Lactic dehydrogenase and glutamic oxalacetic transaminase in anemia. Arch. intern. Med. **102**, 115—123 (1958).

# VIROLOGY MONOGRAPHS

# VIROLOGY
# MONOGRAPHS